Breast Cancer

Breast Cancer

The Facts You Need to Know about
Diagnosis, Treatment and Beyond

Pat Kelly with
Mark Levine MD, MSc, FRCP (C)

FIREFLY BOOKS

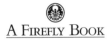

A FIREFLY BOOK

Published by Firefly Books (U.S.) Inc. 2003

First Printing

U.S. CATALOGING IN PUBLICATION DATA

Kelly, Pat
    Breast cancer : the facts you need / Pat Kelly. – 1st ed.

[152] p. : ill. ; cm. (Your personal health)
Includes index.

Summary: A guide for women and their families to understanding what breast cancer is, how it is treated, and how to cope with its physical and emotional effects.

ISBN: 1-55297-738-2 (pbk.)

1. Breast – Cancer – Popular works. 2. Breast cancer – Treatment – Popular works. I. Title. II. Series.

616.99/449 21   RC280.B8.K45 2003

Published in the United States in 2003 by
Firefly Books (U.S.) Inc.
P.O. Box 1338, Ellicott Station
Buffalo, New York, USA
14205

Published in Canada in 2002 by Key Porter Books Limited.

Electronic formatting: Heidi Palfrey
Design: Jack Steiner

Printed and bound in Canada

From the women who shared the stories
of their struggles and rewards.

To all women facing the challenge of
breast cancer and those who care for them:

From knowledge comes strength.

And

To Kate and Kelly Fenn,
my daughters,
and to my beloved Hugh:

Love and hugs,
Mommy Pat

Acknowledgments

We are grateful to the many members of the breast cancer survivor community and to all those who contributed their time to the writing of this book.

If you have any comments about this book, please address them to:

Pat Kelly
PISCES
E-mail: pisces1@on.aibn.com

or visit the PISCES Web site: www.piscesonline.ca.

Contents

Preface

This book is for the thousands of women who have been told, "I'm sorry, but you have breast cancer." It is also for the husbands, lovers, partners, friends, daughters, mothers, colleagues, co-workers, and family members who are trying to help and understand. This book has been written by experts in the field—other women living with breast cancer, women who know the journey from "the inside out"—and the health care team that supports us.

The idea for this book began in Burlington, Ontario, Canada, in 1988. I had been diagnosed with breast cancer in 1987 at the age of thirty-four and later met Barb Sullivan, who had been diagnosed a year earlier, aged forty-three. Each of us was looking for support, information, and encouragement at a time when Canada had no groups, information about treatments was very hard to find, and women didn't talk about cancer because they feared how others might react. Fortunately Barb and I found each other, and we soon realized there were probably other women like us looking for help, so we decided to hold a meeting. In April 1988, we first met at the local YMCA where thirty-five other women from our community joined us. Very quickly the membership grew as other women came to share stories, to give support and information, to cry and to laugh, to mourn together for those who died—and, most importantly, to learn to live *with* cancer. The group that started at the Y continues to meet every month, providing support, information, and advocacy for women and their families affected by breast cancer.

Much has happened since that first meeting. Women now talk openly about having cancer, information is easier to find, and survivors and advocates have made significant gains in the decision making about all aspects of the disease. All across Canada—from Fredericton to Thunder Bay to Regina to Whitehorse—small groups have started with three or four women gathered at kitchen tables, in church basements, or in the waiting rooms of doctors' offices and clinics. More women are taking an active part in their diagnosis, treatment, and healing. Many groups and individuals are organizing advocacy efforts in order to bring about systemic changes in health care at the local, regional, and national levels.

While breast cancer continues to occur at alarmingly high rates, there is important good news. The death rate is finally starting to drop, moderately, in Canada and the United States, particularly in younger, premenopausal women. Clinical practice guidelines, outlining the best way to treat the disease, have now been developed as one way to ensure all women and their doctors understand the range of options. Surgery, radiation, hormones, and chemotherapy are still standard treatments, but newer and more effective forms of some therapies are making a difference in survival rates. There is evidence that support groups, complementary therapies, and mind-body techniques, which encourage wellness, play an important role in the care and quality of life of women with breast cancer.

And there has been another very personal and quite dramatic change over the past fourteen years. Mark Levine and I started our relationship as doctor and patient—and in the beginning we had very different views about the world of breast cancer. Advocacy was not something taught at medical school. We spent a lot of time trying to convince each other that we were right. And, eventually, we were *both* right.

Over the years we have come to value our differences of opinions and to seek one another out—each experts in our own knowledge. We have developed a relationship based upon trust, experience, and friendship.

Today, advocacy is now valued as an integral part of the comprehensive breast cancer team. As Dr. Larry Norton, a respected colleague, once said, "It is an expression of our unity of purpose as humans dedi-cated to the eradication of human suffering. It is the realization that we are all in this together."

We hope our book reflects the heightened awareness about breast cancer and the needs of women now being diagnosed with it. Our intent is that this knowledge will serve to enlighten you—intellectually and spiritually—with honesty and compassion.

In hope and good health,

PAT KELLY AND MARK LEVINE

October 2002

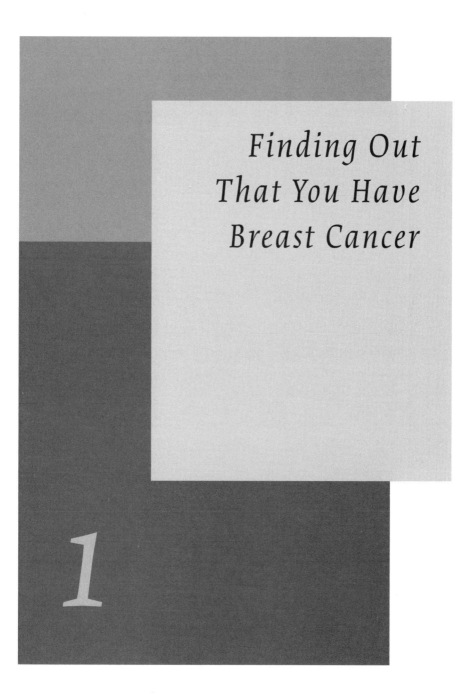

Finding Out
That You Have
Breast Cancer

1

This chapter will help explain some of the most common emotional responses that women talk about when they learn they have breast cancer. It is intended to help you put these feelings into perspective and find what other women have found helpful.

> *I was scared to death I would die and leave my two children alone. Now I can appreciate everything around me, especially my friends and my family. Without my friends I don't know how I would have survived. It has been nine years now and every year I am thankful.*

There Must Be Some Mistake!

Few of us are ready when our fear of cancer becomes a reality. But each year more than 205,000 women in the United States and an additional 18,000 Canadian women learn that they have breast cancer. They are women of all ages and lifestyles; women who believed themselves to be healthy; women we know and care about; women just like us.

> "Beauty and tragedy are inextricably interwoven in people with serious illness. Those with diseases such as cancer can be heroic and frightened, generous and selfish. They can indeed 'live beyond limits.'"
>
> —DR. DAVID SPIEGEL,
> *Living beyond Limits: New Hope and Help for Facing Life-Threatening Illness*

Very few people truly understand what you're going through as a
cancer patient. They care and they try to understand, but unless they've
been there themselves, they really can't.

I think the most important goal is to provide those of us undergoing
treatment some hope that we will recover, survive, and perhaps even
be cured. I am well enough aware of the severity of my illness not to
fool myself that all is well. But the nurses, volunteers, and alternative
practitioners that I have dealt with seem far more aware than my doctors
of the power of language to effect empowerment in people.

If you have just learned that you have breast cancer, you may feel
overwhelmed and unable to decide what to do next. You may be
frightened. You may feel lonely. These feelings are very, very common
for newly diagnosed women. *You are not alone. You are not helpless.* Over a
million women living with breast cancer in North America prove these
truths each and every day. There are people who can help you cope.
There is information that can help you make the right decisions for
you. There is support for who you are now and what you must do.

Now may be a time to cry, to grieve, and to be angry. But it is also a
time to care for yourself. Soon you will be able to plan your treatments
and to begin to heal.

One of the joys of surviving cancer has been the strengthened bond
between myself and my husband and my children. We are kinder to
each other now, realizing that there is no time for harsh words, no time
to be wasted. Sometimes we cling together for a brief moment, sharing
unspeakable thoughts in a terrifying, yet richly comforting way.

As you begin to try to understand what it will be like for you to
have cancer, you may find it helpful to think about living with cancer
as a journey. Like any other journey, you can plan, but you cannot be

certain where your trip will lead you, when you will arrive, or what you will find along the way. What lies ahead for you will be both good and bad. You will meet fellow travelers, learn to watch the view, tolerate the delays, and look forward to (or dread) the stops along the way.

You can begin your journey by replacing your fear about what might be ahead with information you can use in the here and now.

> *I was devastated and very sad. I realized that all the crap I had been ignoring needed looking at. I'm still on the journey and will always be recovering. After much counseling, marital and personal, my life is good. I'm learning to be real to others and myself. I'm listening to my body and respecting what it is telling me. I'm giving different messages to my three daughters—we are all feminists working to bring dignity, respect, and safety to all women, children, and men.*

The Emotional Side of Cancer

When you learn that you have breast cancer, you may feel very alone or frightened. Some of us wonder if we are going crazy. We aren't. Cancer is a major life crisis. While you are in a crisis, you can expect to feel confused and emotional. Here are some of the emotions that breast cancer survivors remember from the time of their own diagnosis and in the months that followed. Some of these feelings may be familiar to you.

> *Throughout my treatment I felt I was being cared for quite well. My only complaint was that, other than a brief visit from a support group member, I felt very alone. If it weren't for my hospital roommate, it would have been terrifying. We have maintained our friendship and have a bond that no one who hasn't had cancer would have.*

FEAR

Fear of death. Fear of what life will be—can be—now. Fear of loss of strength, health, femininity, sexual attractiveness, and vigor. Fear of being diminished, of aging sooner than your time. Fear both for yourself and for your family and friends.

> *The initial diagnosis was traumatic for me. I was thirty-six years old, single, with a child. I was very scared. What would it be like? Was I going to die? After I got over the shock and everything settled down, the experience became very positive because it forced me to make changes in my life that I was putting off. I moved from where I was living, I made physical changes about how I looked, and I joined a Nautilus program. It made me realize how precious life is, and I'm much happier than I was before. When they did an ultrasound and thought the cancer had spread, I thought I was dying. But it hadn't. Now I'm just happy to be alive. Life is less scary when you have had cancer. Nothing is worse.*

SHOCK AND DENIAL

You may be thinking, "This just can't be happening. I took good care of myself. I didn't smoke. I ate (mostly) healthy foods. I exercised. I handled the stress in my life. Nobody in my family has had breast cancer. So how could I have cancer?" The first reaction may be a temporary state of shock from which we gradually recuperate. When the initial feeling of numbness begins to disappear and we begin to collect our thoughts the usual response is, "No, it can't be true." Since we all, unconsciously, think we are immortal, it is unimaginable to face a possibility of death. Gradually, you will find yourself adjusting to the reality of diagnosis and decision making.

ANGER

Like many of us, you may be very angry that this disease has happened to you. Perhaps you found a lump or some change in your breast a while ago and didn't do anything about it. Or you discovered changes many months ago and your doctor said, "Let's just wait and see." Or you didn't go back to see your doctor. Now it's cancer. Anger at yourself or others is understandable and may be justifiable. But anger can also prevent you from making decisions or can get in the way of relationships with people you may need to depend upon.

GUILT

Many women feel guilty about things they did or didn't do that they believe may have caused their cancer. *Always remember that you didn't do anything to cause the cancer.* The majority of women diagnosed with breast cancer have none of the known risk factors, other than age. There is probably no single cause of this disease. It just happened and no one can say for sure why it has happened to you. Learning to live with this uncertainty is one of the greatest challenges for women with breast cancer.

HOPELESSNESS/HELPLESSNESS

You may feel that your health is gone forever. You may even think your life is over. Overnight you have been transformed from a healthy, productive woman to someone you don't know, someone who is terribly ill and may, even now, be dying. You may feel hopeless and helpless, a cancer patient whose future is locked in place by this illness. You may, in your darkest moments, wish you could die quickly and painlessly right now and not have to face the uncertainty of the months ahead.

> *After my diagnosis, I had to stop working for the first time in my life. The debilitating treatments I was receiving made me dependent on my family and friends, which, being a very dynamic, active, and independent person, I had difficulty accepting.*

ACCEPTING YOUR EMOTIONS

No one can say how long the ups and downs and the emotional grieving will continue. For some women, this period of uncertainty and confusion can last long after the end of their treatment.

> *I am envious of women who feel totally cured. I may not have cancer, but cancer certainly has me. I always feel like it's a lurking danger, like we're legally separated but can never be divorced. I live more on the edge now. I take risks that perhaps I shouldn't take and would never have taken before.*

There will always be sadness for the losses, grief, and longing for what might have been a more carefree life. Those feelings eventually fade for most women. Cancer can be a turning point in your life. For now, try to remember that dramatic mood swings are to be expected. They are part of learning to be a cancer survivor. You may keep coming back to these emotions as you learn to live with cancer and go from being a patient to a woman whose life has been challenged by cancer.

"I wonder if I will ever make plans again?

Life goes on around me. I am aware of it, but not involved. I am unto myself. Tears are close, always.

Today I need to work. To have another identity besides 'patient.' I am tired. But I must fight. Say no to this intrusion. Not lay down my will.

This is the last exercise class with a real breast. Next time I'll have to worry about my socks falling out.

How do you say goodbye to a breast? I've had it for forty-five years. I think I'll miss it. But I'm playing it cool.

The cancer lady comes. Shows me her wares. Great flopping prosthesis. I think yuck! I am not interested right now. She says, *"Don't carry your purse on your affected side and always wear your gloves when gardening!"* May she strangle in her knickers.

It is more complicated than I thought. I wasn't going to be bothered by losing a breast. I am. I don't like how I look. I look amputated. I am different. I am a cancer patient. Will I ever be unaware of my chest?

Did you know you can't cry while laying on your back? You get water in your ears.

A large sign says Cancer Clinic. I am identified even before I enter. I want to go in disguise. I do not belong here. I think I will leave.

It is a sit-on-the-edge-of-your-seat kind of place. Scary. At the mercy of machines. All supposed to do a job. But do they?

Tell me again that I'll be fine. Give me hope to grow with. Words to recover by."

—BARB SULLIVAN,
My Broken Breast Book

Many women find that support groups are very helpful in dealing with the emotional side of cancer. At a support group, you can expect to meet other women who are living with breast cancer. Some members are newly diagnosed, others will still be coming to the group years after treatments have ended. You can talk about your fears or relationships, or you may just want to sit quietly and listen. But, most importantly, you meet other women who know about living with breast cancer. They can offer support and education, even laughter and warm hugs, along with hope.

Support groups aren't for everyone; in fact, many women find all the comfort and support they need among friends and family. Again, consider groups as one option to explore, not a requirement for everyone.

SUMMARY

As you will have realized by now, cancer is as much an emotional and psychological experience as it is physical. Feeling hurt, angry, or confused is normal. And your family and friends may share some of these worries and feelings with you. Everyone who cares about you will be looking to you to give them a signal; let them know if you want to talk (or don't want to talk) and how they can help.

Support groups can also help. The best groups work in the following ways:

- by listening to each other and sharing personal stories
- by sharing information based on personal experiences
- by offering emotional support through sympathy and understanding
- by providing a sense of belonging

Whether you choose to seek support from a group or from family and friends, the goal is the same: to gain control, to help make choices, to help you feel hopeful, and to help you overcome loneliness.

Remember that you have control over the choices you make and *how* you choose to make this journey through cancer territory. Like many other women, you may also find meaningful and rewarding surprises along the way to healing.

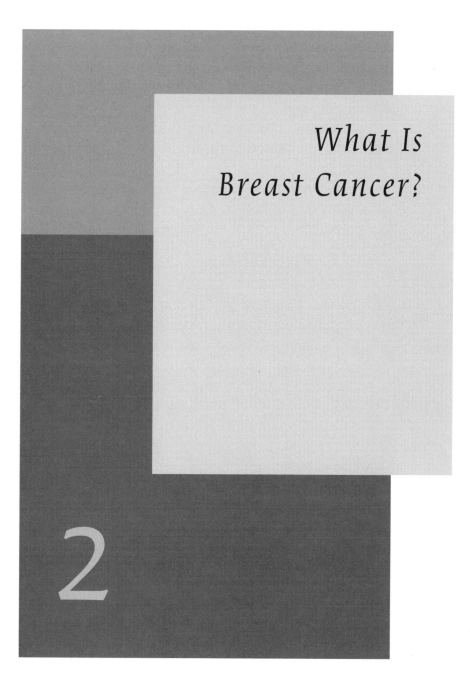

What Is
Breast Cancer?

2

This chapter will explain what breast cancer is. It will also explore some of the risk factors for breast cancer, and why some women are more likely to get it than others. As you will see, risk factors really don't help explain why most women develop breast cancer. There is still much that is unknown about the cause of this disease.

Women need to know that they can and should have a part in all of the decision making regarding their diagnosis.

A Life-Changing Disease

Breast cancer is the unregulated growth of abnormal cells in the breast. In North America, it is the most common type of cancer in women and one of the most treatable types. Breast cancer threatens and changes our lives. Our bodies and our relationships with others can be forever altered. This disease, like other life-threatening diseases, can bring with it fear, confusion, pain, and isolation. Cancer forces us to make difficult choices at a time when we are feeling shocked and confused.

HOW DOES BREAST CANCER START?

Like all forms of cancer, breast cancer starts in one cell. Cells are the smallest structural unit of living matter that can function independently in the body. They are the building blocks of our bodies. Healthy cells grow at a normal rate. Cancer cells grow at an accelerated rate and continue to grow until they crowd out the normal cells. Unlike normal cells, cancer cells don't know how to turn off their growth. The abnormal growth rate is caused by changes or mutations in the genetic material inside the cell. These mutations may be inherited from our parents or caused by exposure to a mutating substance. It usually takes more than one "hit" of exposure to a cancer-causing substance to cause changes. Cancerous tumors or lumps contain mutated as well as normal cells.

IS ALL BREAST CANCER THE SAME?

In one word, no. There are several kinds of breast cancer, depending on where in the breast tissue the tumor starts to grow. About one-half of all breast cancer tumors are first found in the upper, outer part of the breast, but they can appear anywhere in the breast tissue. Each breast has fifteen to twenty sections, called "lobes," which have many smaller sections, called "lobules." Thin tubes, called "ducts," connect the lobes and lobules (see Figure 2.1). The lobes, lobules, and ducts make and secrete milk for breast-feeding. Eighty-five percent of breast cancers start in the ducts, 12 percent in the lobules, and the remaining 2 percent start in the surrounding tissue. Not all breast cancers are found in the form of a lump. Other changes that can indicate cancer are dimpling around the nipple, secretions or fluid leaking from the nipple, and changes in the skin texture that may make it look like the skin of an orange, called "peau d'orange."

Carcinoma in Situ

"In situ" means the cancer is confined to the ducts or lobules and has not spread to the surrounding fatty tissue. Because it has not invaded the surrounding tissue, it is not truly a cancer.

Lobular Carcinoma in Situ (LCIS)   This is a type of non-invasive tumor that begins in the lobules but does not spread through their walls. It is very rare. Most cancer specialists feel that LCIS does not develop into invasive cancer. However women with LCIS are at higher risk of developing invasive breast cancer in both breasts compared to the normal population

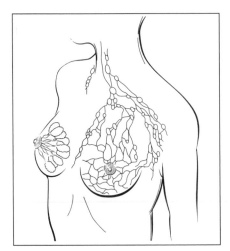

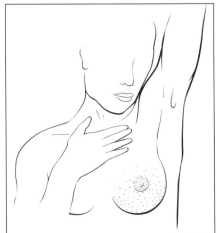

FIGURE 2.1 *Cross-section of breast showing the network of milk-producing lobes connected by thin tubes or ducts*

FIGURE 2.2 *Inflammatory breast cancer (peau d'orange)*

Ductal Carcinoma in Situ (DCIS)   This is a very common type of non-invasive tumor that does not spread outside the duct walls. Some specialists think more women die *with* DCIS than *because* of it. Thirty years ago DCIS was diagnosed in about 6 percent of patients. Today, about 20 percent of patients are diagnosed with DCIS, probably due to advances in early detection through mammography. Treatment is usually surgery and radiation.

Infiltrating Ductal Carcinoma (IDC)

This type of breast cancer starts inside the cells of the milk ducts and invades outside the duct walls into the surrounding tissue. Over time, it may also spread through the lymph system or bloodstream to other organs or bones. Infiltrating ductal carcinoma accounts for about 85 percent of all breast cancers.

Infiltrating Lobular Carcinoma (ILC)

Lobular carcinoma starts in the lobes of the breast and, like ductal carcinoma, it can spread to other parts of the body through blood or the lymph system. About 12 percent of breast cancers start in the lobules or lobes.

Inflammatory Breast Cancer (IBC)

This is an uncommon type of breast cancer that can cause redness, swelling, and an increase in skin temperature (Figure 2.2). The cancer cells in inflammatory breast cancer are located in the lymph vessels of the skin, growing in sheets rather than as a solid tumor. The cancer cells block the lymphatic channels and cause swelling of the skin of the breast. It can often be found spread throughout the breast with no solid tumor or palpable mass. There can be increased breast density compared with previous mammograms, which should be considered a suspicious finding. One or more of the following symptoms may be caused by IBC:

+ Swelling, itching, bruising, or thickening of skin, usually sudden, sometimes a cup size in a few days
+ Pink, red, or dark colored area of skin, sometimes textured like an orange (peau d'orange)
+ Nipple retraction, discharge, or change in color and texture
+ Breast is hot or warm to the touch
+ Breast pain (throbbing, constant ache to stabbing pains)

Paget's Disease

Paget's disease (Figure 2.3) shows up as itching and scaling of the nipple that doesn't get better. The cancer cells are in the skin of the nipples. Sometimes there is cancer inside the breast tissue as well.

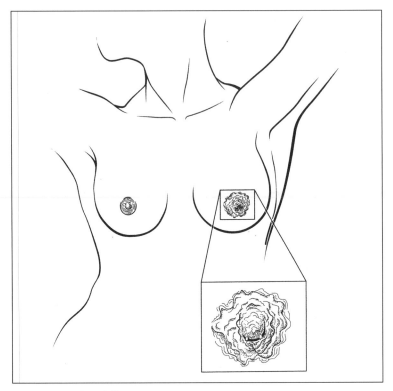

FIGURE 2.3   *Paget's disease*

How Does Cancer Spread Outside the Breast?

Cancer cells can break off from the tumor and travel through blood vessels or lymph fluid to other organs and bones. When you are diagnosed with breast cancer, and before you begin treatment, your doctors will examine you and perform tests, x-rays, and scans that will help to determine if your cancer has spread beyond the breast to lymph tissue or to other organs.

How Fast Does Breast Cancer Grow?

Most breast cancers grow slowly, which is helpful to remember when you are trying to make treatment decisions (Figure 2.4). Although it can

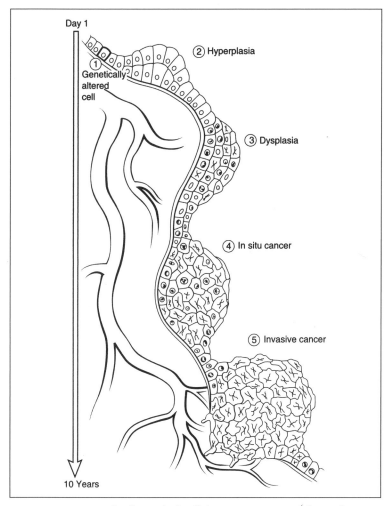

FIGURE 2.4 *Progression from a single cell change to tumor mass (please refer to Glossary for explanation of terms)*

be difficult to wait for your test results so you can make treatment decisions, you do have time to learn about your type of breast cancer and carefully consider which options will be best for you. The average doubling time of a breast cell is 100 days. It takes approximately a billion cells to form a breast tumor 1 cm in size, which means that, on average, most cancers have been around for six to ten years before they can be felt as a lump or seen on a mammogram. Some cancers grow quickly, while others grow slowly—growing, resting, and then growing again. How fast a tumor grows varies from one person to the next.

Why Is Cancer So Hard to Treat or Cure?

Cancer is not something that invades our body from the outside like a virus or bacteria; cancer is not like an injury or trauma. Cancer is a disease of the self: the body's own cells change and grow out of control. This is why it is so hard to stop cancer cells from growing without also harming healthy cells.

> *Our main goal in society should be to find a way to kill cancer cells. All money should go to this goal, since with a cure, the need for many other services would be eliminated. Effective research is the key to a cure for cancer. We can put people on the moon—why can't we kill a cancer cell?*

Who Gets Breast Cancer?

This section will explain some of the risk factors for breast cancer, and why some women are more likely to get it than others. As you will see, risk factors really don't explain why some women develop breast cancer. Much is still unknown about the causes of this disease.

Why Did This Happen to Me?

What is the most important breast cancer risk factor? Simply being a woman.

Many women who have just learned of their condition wonder what they might have done to cause the disease. No one can tell you exactly what caused your body to develop breast cancer. The known risk factors are not very helpful in understanding why some women get the disease. Not everyone who has a high risk factor will get the disease. Many women who are diagnosed have none of the risk factors. The effects of risk factors are modest at best.

For example, if having a family history increases the risk somewhere between one-and-a-half and twofold, then for a forty-year-old woman the annual risk of getting breast cancer in the next five years would increase from 1 in 1,000 to 2 in 1,000. As you can see, even when the risk is doubled, the chances of getting cancer are still very small.

Simply because we are women, and our bodies produce hormones and we develop breasts, we are all at risk for breast cancer. There is also a risk for men, though it is much smaller: about 1 in every 100 breast cancer cases are diagnosed in men.

Seventy percent of women with breast cancer have none of the known risk factors, other than age. Risk factors are based on the information and statistics gathered from large groups of women. Other than inherited gene mutations, the effect of any specific risk factor for any individual woman is small. Even when your risk factors are known, no one can predict what will happen to any one woman in particular.

The Causes of Breast Cancer

There is probably no single cause of this disease. Researchers have found that several different factors working together appear to increase the risk of breast cancer. The ways in which different risk factors interact with each other is not fully understood. Because of their genetic history, their lifestyles, and what they are exposed to in their lifetime, some women are more likely to get the disease than others. The incidence of breast cancer is higher in industrialized countries such as Canada, Northern Europe, and the United States than in other parts of the world.

The following factors may increase your risk for breast cancer.

Age

The risk of developing breast cancer increases as a woman grows older. For example, the annual risk of a woman getting breast cancer increases dramatically between the ages of forty and fifty. It increases again by age seventy. In one year, out of 100,000 women between the ages forty and forty-four, 90 will get breast cancer. For women aged seventy to seventy-four, 310 out of 100,000 will get the disease in one year. Two-thirds of breast cancers are diagnosed in women over the age of fifty.

For a woman born today, her risk by age thirty is 1 in 2,000. One in nine Canadian women will be diagnosed with breast cancer before age 85 (see Figure 2.5).

By age 40:	1 out of 233
By age 50:	1 out of 53
By age 60:	1 out of 22
By age 70:	1 out of 13
By age 80:	1 out of 9

SOURCE: *NCI SEER Program, 1995–1997*

Personal and Family History/Genetics

If you have already had breast cancer, or a close family member was diagnosed with breast cancer before she reached menopause, you are at greater risk. For example, if your mother had breast cancer before age forty, then your risk of developing this disease is doubled. And if you have many other close relatives with breast cancer your risk may be much higher.

Recent research shows that some women with breast cancer have inherited a mutated gene linked to the development of breast and ovarian cancer (BRCA1) or breast cancer (BRCA2) (see Figures 2.6 and 2.7).

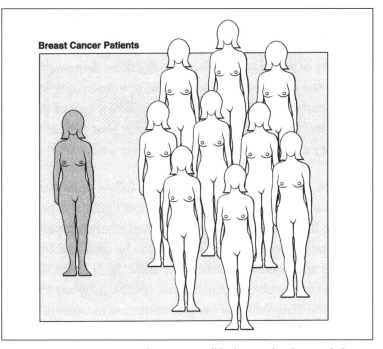

FIGURE 2.5 *One in nine Canadian women will be diagnosed with cancer before age 85. You are not alone.*

Factors that should raise your suspicion include early onset of disease (before age thirty-five), family history (on either side) of diagnoses in every generation, and linkage with ovarian cancer.

However, if both you and a close family member develop breast cancer, it is not necessarily because you both carry the same gene. The field of research on genetics and breast cancer is relatively new. Discoveries are being made quite rapidly in the area.

A mutant BRCA1 gene on chromosome 17 is probably responsible for about 2 percent of the 18,000 cases of breast cancer diagnosed each year. In Canada, as many as one-quarter of the cases occur in women aged forty-five and younger. A mutant BRCA1 gene is found in nearly half of the

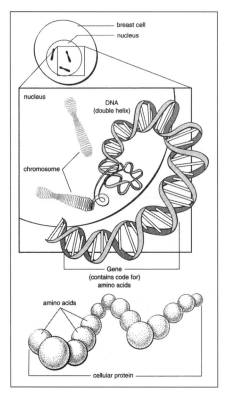

FIGURE 2.6   *DNA, which carries the instructions that allow cells to make proteins, is made up of four chemical bases. Tightly coiled strands of DNA are packaged in units called chromosomes, housed in the cell's nucleus. Working subunits of DNA are known as genes.*

families with high incidence of breast cancer and in at least 80 percent of the families with a history of both early onset breast cancer and ovarian cancer.

However, most diseases and traits don't follow simple patterns of inheritance; a variety of factors influence how a gene will perform. Genes come in pairs, with one part inherited from each parent. The BRCA1 susceptibility gene can be inherited from either parent. But even if you have this gene, your risk of disease by age sixty-five is 60 percent, not 100 percent.

There are counseling programs available for anyone who may have an inherited risk for cancer, and your family doctor should be able to tell you where your nearest counseling center is located. You can also contact the American Cancer Society (1-800-ACS-2345) or, in Canada, the Cancer Information Service (1-888-939-3333) about your local services.

Reproductive History

The following factors related to your reproductive history can increase risk:

- Having your first period before age twelve
- Having no children
- Having your first child after age thirty

- Starting menopause after age fifty-five
- Taking hormone replacement therapy (HRT) for symptoms of menopause

Age at the start of your first period   Girls who start menstruating before age twelve appear to be at higher risk than girls who start at an older age. The reason may be that hormones such as estrogen, which are increased when a girl begins having periods, contribute to developing breast cancer. The longer a woman has periods, the greater the exposure to estrogen.

Age at the birth of your first child   Women who have never delivered a child are at higher risk than those who have. Women who have had a first birth after age thirty are at greater risk than women who have had children before thirty. The reason may be that an early pregnancy causes protective changes in the breast tissue, causing the breast cell to mature in some way that differs from the changes that occur later in life.

Age at the start of your menopause   Women who begin menopause later than average (older than forty-five) are at a higher risk for getting breast cancer than women who start earlier. Again, the reason may be that the later menopause begins, the longer the woman is exposed to increased hormone levels associated with having her regular periods.

Hormone replacement therapy (HRT)   Hormone replacement therapy refers to treatment with pills or skin patches that contain estrogen or estrogen and progesterone combined. Hormones are chemicals that affect the activity of certain cells and organs. Both estrogen and progesterone play an important role in a woman's life, regulating menstrual periods and affecting the growth of breast tissue. The ovaries produce these particular hormones, but they can also be made in a laboratory or obtained from plants and animals.

As women leave their childbearing years behind, they begin to produce less estrogen and progesterone. A lack of estrogen can lead to unpleasant menopausal symptoms such as hot flashes and vaginal dryness. It can also contribute to osteoporosis—the loss of bone tissue. HRT is often prescribed to relieve menopausal symptoms and was thought to reduce the risk of osteoporosis. HRT may also be prescribed when a woman experiences premature menopause, whether naturally or as the result of medical treatment. Recent findings about the benefits of HRT suggest HRT be used cautiously and for a shorter duration. HRT is associated with a twofold increase in breast cancer risk, and, as a result, should not be used for women who have had breast cancer.

If you are having problems with menopausal symptoms and are thinking about taking herbal supplements to relieve the discomfort of mood swings, vaginal dryness, night sweats, or other problems, discuss this first with a pharmacist. Some herbal supplements contain natural source estrogens—but these are still estrogens and can affect breast cancer risk and recurrence the same as other forms of hormone replacement therapy.

Abortion and Breast Cancer

A 2002 position paper developed by the U.S. National Breast Cancer Coalition stated that, "The effects of abortion on breast cancer risk may be similar to those of full-term pregnancy, i.e., they may be transient and weaken with age. In other words, there is only very weak and inconclusive data about the link between abortion and breast cancer. This suggests *no* conclusions can reasonably be drawn. Clearly, there is much more we need to learn about the hormonal effects of pregnancy and abortion on breast cancer risk."

A large, 2001 study from Denmark has provided very strong data that induced abortions have no effect on the risk of breast cancer. Also,

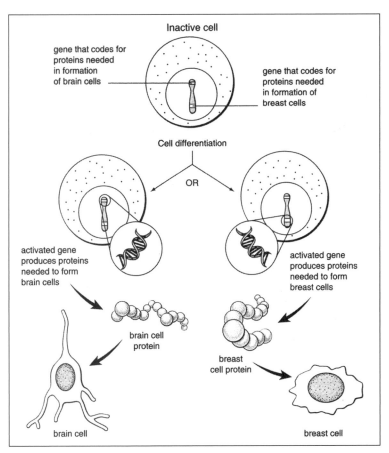

FIGURE 2.7   *Different genes are activated in different cells, creating the specific proteins that program a particular type of cell to develop.*

there is no evidence of a direct relationship between breast cancer and spontaneous abortion (miscarriage) in most of the studies that have been published.

Abortion is one of the most controversial and poorly understood risk factors for breast cancer. A few studies have shown a slight increase, while other studies failed to show any increase.

Breast Implants

Silicone breast implants can cause scar tissue in the breast, but implants do not increase breast cancer risk. When having a mammogram you should let the mammography technologists know if you have implants. X-ray pictures called "implant displacement views" can be used to completely examine the breast tissue.

Birth Control Pills

The hormones that our bodies produce play a role in the development of breast cancer. This is why the age at which we start menstruating, have (or don't have) children, and go through menopause can all influence whether we are at risk. More and more researchers are also focusing on the relationship between breast cancer and other hormones, including those to which we are exposed in the environment and those that we may take in the form of birth control pills. Some studies show that taking birth control pills for more than five years may put us at a higher risk for breast cancer, while others indicate no link. The research is far from conclusive.

Obesity

Being 40 percent above the ideal body weight greatly increases a person's risk of certain types of cancers. Because estrogen—a hormone that has been linked to breast cancer development—is stored in fatty or "adipose" tissue, the more fat we have, the more estrogen is available to influence our endocrine systems and breast tissue.

The extent to which a woman is overweight at the time of her diagnosis may influence the chance of getting breast cancer again. Many women consider a healthy diet and exercise an important part of healing, recovery, and maintaining well-being.

Diet/Nutrition

The total number of calories and the amount of fat you eat on a regular basis may influence your risk for breast cancer. However, there has not been extensive research on individual women to prove this. More and more, we hear of the importance of eating a varied and well-balanced diet, emphasizing fruits and vegetables, low fat, high-fiber foods, and increasing physical activity. In addition, some researchers have found that certain vitamins (such as A, C, and E) and selenium, which are also known as antioxidants, may help to prevent cancer.

Drinking alcohol can also be a risk factor. Researches have found that a moderate intake (3 oz per day) may increase one's risk of developing breast cancer.

Environmental Factors

The study of links between elements in the environment and the development of breast cancer is slowly getting attention. Many elements that women are exposed to over their lifetime are being researched for their possible link to breast cancer. These include pesticides, chlorine-based "organochlorines" (which contain such toxins such as PCBs, dioxin, and DDT), and hazardous wastes such as chrome, mercury, and other heavy metals and chemicals.

A report of the Ontario Task Force on the Primary Prevention of Cancer (March 1991) pointed out numerous research studies that have examined the link between breast cancer and toxic substances in the environment. After examining the issue, the Task Force produced a series of strong recommendations relating to environmental hazards. Similarly strong recommendations were put forward in 1994 by the International Joint Commission on the Great Lakes after its examination of the effect of Great Lakes water on human health.

On the other hand, a study reported in the October 30, 1997, issue of the *New England Journal of Medicine* presented the strongest evidence to date that pesticides do not cause breast cancer. Whether there are other chemicals associated with cancer remains untested, but the results of this study show no association to DDT and PCBs, the most common environmental chemicals blamed for cancer.

As with most of the suspected causes of breast cancer, more research is needed.

Exposure to Radiation

Researchers studied a large population of women who were exposed to radiation at a young age, such as that from the atom bomb at Hiroshima and Nagasaki, and girls who had tuberculosis at a young age whose treatment involved getting frequent x-rays. (Note that these were doses of radiation much, much higher than what we receive today from a mammogram.) Exposure to radiation at a young age (up to age thirty or thirty-five) has been shown to increase the risk of breast cancer throughout life, particularly if it was given to the chest. The researchers found that radiation exposure at older ages has little effect on developing breast cancer.

WHAT DOESN'T CAUSE BREAST CANCER

There is no reason to believe that fondling, bumping, or injuring the breasts can cause cancer. Breast cancer is not contagious, and it cannot be transmitted from one person to another. Some women who have breast cancer worry that their stressful lifestyle caused the cancer to develop. There is currently no evidence-based research showing that stress contributes to cancer development.

SUMMARY

It appears that breast cells may be very sensitive to radiation, diet, hormonal changes, pregnancy, and environmental toxins during adolescence and the early teen years. This sensitivity may result in cellular changes, which can increase or decrease the likelihood of developing breast cancer later in life. Today, we don't have much control over these factors.

Most women with breast cancer have none of the known risk factors for their age. However, exposure to the hormone estrogen is likely a determining factor.

No one can tell you exactly what happened to cause you to develop breast cancer. But you do have control over your treatment choices and what you do to help yourself to become well again.

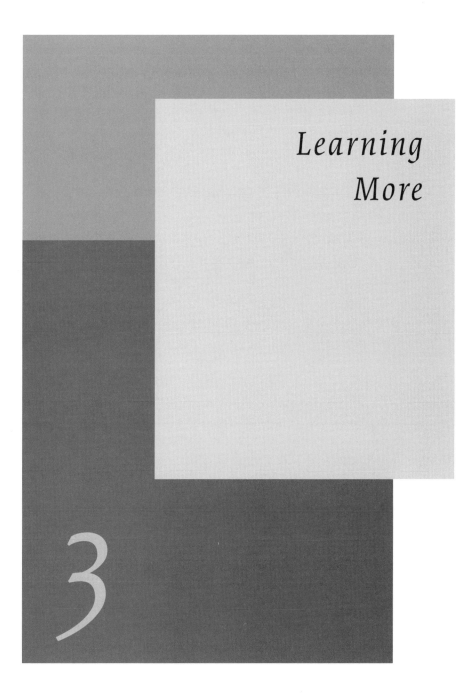

Learning More

3

This chapter explains basic information about the different types of breast cancer, to help you start to understand the disease.

Forget the cookies and coffee, give me information, get me support, let me make an informed decision.

What Can My Doctor Tell Me about My Breast Cancer?

The first step in deciding which treatment is right for you is to understand as much as you can about *your* tumor. The following tests are commonly used to diagnose your cancer, determine the extent of the disease, and help you understand which treatments are right for your type of cancer.

BIOPSY

When your cancer was diagnosed, some tissue was removed from your breast so it could be analyzed. Often, as a first step in diagnosing a lump, a physician will insert a small needle into the lump and aspirate some cells. These cells are then sent to a laboratory for examination under a microscope. This is called "aspiration cytology" and should not be confused with a biopsy. If the lump is suspected to be a cyst (a small harmless sac of fluid), an ultrasound exam or a technique called "fine-needle aspirate" can help confirm it. If the fluid drawn out by the fine needle aspirate is bloody, it will be sent for testing. If it is not, the lump is just a cyst and no further testing need be done. The lump will go away once the fluid is removed.

A biopsy involves the actual removal of a piece of tissue (involving many hundreds of cells) from the breast. Types of biopsies include inserting a long needle into the side of the lump (a "core biopsy" or

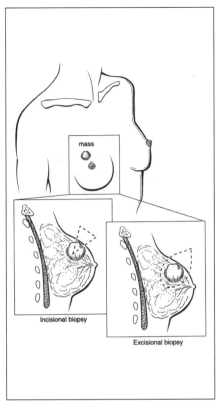

FIGURE 3.1 *Incisional and excisional biopsy*

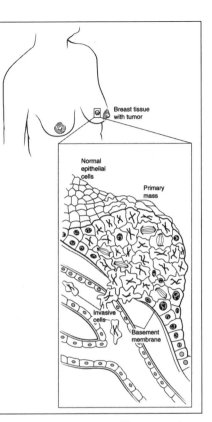

FIGURE 3.2 *Invasive or infiltrating carcinoma, showing that the tumor has broken through the basement membrane and cells are shed into the blood and lymph system*

"incisional biopsy," see Figure 3.1) or cutting out the lump through surgery ("excisional biopsy"). A pathologist will examine the tissue that was removed and write a report about what he or she found. Details about the tumor's appearance help provide information about the type of breast cancer. This information will be helpful in planning your treatment. The pathologist also examines and describes the features of the cancer in detail so a prognosis can be made about the possible future outcome of treatments.

THE PATHOLOGY REPORT

The pathology report should indicate the size of the tumor (1 cm, 2 cm, 3 cm, etc.) and whether or not the cancer cells are spreading. Cancer that is spreading, also known as "invasive cancer" or "infiltrating cancer," has grown outside the basement membrane of the cells and into the surrounding tissue (Figure 3.2). This is different from a condition known as "carcinoma in situ," which is not cancerous but may indicate that cancer could develop.

The following factors will indicate the seriousness of the disease:

+ the number (if any) of lymph nodes involved
+ the size of the tumor at the time of diagnosis
+ the grade of the tumor (grade means wild-looking or aggressive cells)
+ the extent to which the cancer cells are spreading into the surrounding tissue
+ whether the tumor is highly sensitive to the influence of hormones

Axillary Lymph Nodes

After you have had the surgery to treat the breast cancer, the pathologist will examine the breast tissue and the lymph nodes from the armpit that were removed. There are approximately twenty-five to sixty lymph nodes under each arm, and some of these will have been removed at the time of your surgery and examined under the microscope. At least ten nodes should be examined. If the nodes contain cancer cells (this is called being "node-positive"), it is likely that cancer cells have spread to other parts of the body. The number of lymph nodes, if any, involved with the tumor is one of the most important factors in determining prognosis. (See Chapter 4 for more information.)

Histologic Grade

Once the pathologist has determined what kind of breast cancer you have, he or she will then look more closely at the characteristics and

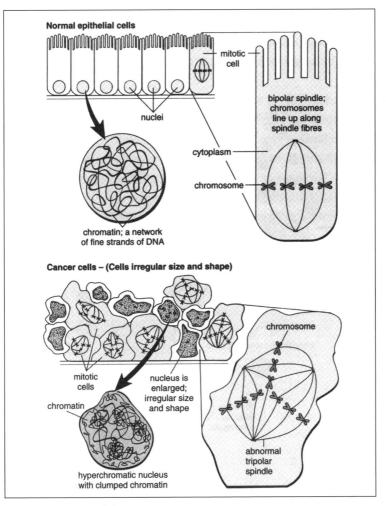

FIGURE 3.3 *How cells become cancerous*

"activity" of the tumor cells. This is described as the "histologic grade." They sometimes refer to the tumors as being "wild-looking" or poorly differentiated, meaning the tumor growth is very active and the cancer cells look very different from normal breast cells. Odd-shaped, wild-looking, or unusual-looking cells are thought to be more aggressive

(Figure 3.3). Cells that look closer to normal (called well-differentiated) are usually less aggressive. The pathologist will also look for how many and how quickly cells are dividing. The most aggressive cancers tend to have many cells dividing at the same time, growing more rapidly. Less aggressive cancers tend to have very few dividing cells.

Nuclear Grade

"Nuclear grade" is another indicator pathologists use. It measures the size of the cell nucleus and the pattern of chromosome material.

Lymphatic-Vascular Invasion

The pathologist will also look to see if there are any cancer cells in the middle of the blood vessels or lymph vessels in the breast tissue. When cancer cells are found here, the cancer is also in the lymph system.

Estrogen Receptor Test and Progesterone Receptor Test

Pathologists perform other tests on the tissue or tumor that was removed from your breast. The tests conducted will vary depending on your hospital and in which province or state you live. Two tests that determine whether the tumor is sensitive to certain hormones are the Estrogen Receptor (ER) Test and the Progesterone Receptor (PR) Test. If the tumors have binding or docking sites on the surface of their cells where the hormone proteins can attach and cause changes in the cell growth, we say they are estrogen receptor positive or progesterone receptor positive (see Figure 3.4).

Usually, tumors in women who have already been through menopause are estrogen receptor positive and those in premenopausal women are estrogen receptor negative, but this isn't always true. Measuring ER and PR is important for two reasons. The results could be prognostic: generally ER-negative tumors are more aggressive. The results can also be predictive of response to treatment. ER-positive

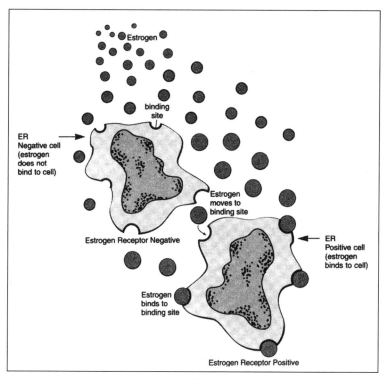

FIGURE 3.4   *Estrogen receptor positive cell and estrogen receptor negative cell*

tumors can be treated with anti-estrogen drugs such as tamoxifen or aromatose inhibitors.

> *One improvement that needs to be made is the waiting time between tests and diagnosis. It is hard to feel optimistic when you don't know what you're facing.*

FLOW CYTOMETRY AND S-PHASE FRACTION ACTIVITY TESTS

Other tests that are sometimes used to measure the activity level of tumor cells are the flow cytometry test and the S-phase fraction activity test. Breast cancer's "S-phase fraction" (SPF) is the percentage of cancer cells replicating their DNA. DNA replication usually signals that a cell is getting ready to split into two new cells. A low SPF indicates the cancer is growing fairly slowly and a high SPF shows the cell is growing rapidly. Rapidly growing tumors need to be treated with more aggressive treatments than those that grow slowly.

Whether these tests add any significant new information compared to older tests in predicting how a woman's breast cancer develops is questionable.

HER-2/neu Oncogene

Other tests include measures of HER-2/neu oncogene. Oncogenes are genes that lead to cancer or cancer growth (Figure 3.5). About 25 percent of breast cancer patients appear to have a great deal of HER-2/neu oncogene material. This gene may be associated with a more active or aggressive disease. A new drug called trastuzumab (Herceptin) acts against tumors that overexpress HER-2/neu. This agent is currently used in situations where the cancer has spread or "metastasized." The gene tests to determine HER-2/neu are performed on a portion of the biopsy specimen.

Tests That May Be Used to Determine If Cancer Has Spread

Bone Scans

This is an imaging method that indicates if the cancer has spread to bone tissue. A small amount of radioactive dye is injected into a vein, which is then carried throughout your system. In places where there is a cancerous tumor in the bone, the radioactive dye will accumulate and the image will indicate an abnormality is present. The radioactive particles will not harm you or cause the cancer to grow.

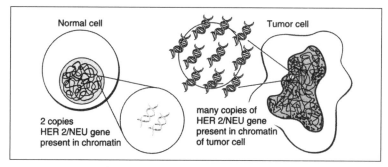

FIGURE 3.5   *Normal and overexpression of HER-2/neu oncogene*

Ultrasound

This is an imaging method commonly used to examine the liver. Sound waves are bounced off the liver to create a picture.

Computerized Axial Tomography (CAT) Scans

In this test, a computer takes multiple x-rays from many different angles and combines them to create a cross-sectional picture of the internal organs. CAT scans are painless and are usually performed in the x-ray department of hospitals. They can detect the spread of disease to internal organs like the liver.

Magnetic Resonance Imaging (MRI) Scans

Another painless method of imaging is the MRI. MRI scans use radio waves and magnets that are painlessly directed through your body to produce detailed images of internal organs.

How Can I Know What Stage My Cancer Is At?

Staging is the process of finding out how much cancer there is in your body and where it is located. Knowing the stage of your cancer will help your doctor determine your prognosis and suggest the most effective treatments for you. Staging is determined by the following:

+ the size of your tumor
+ whether lymph nodes are involved and, if so, how many
+ indications of metastasis or spread of the cancer cells beyond the breast tissue and axillary nodes at the time of diagnosis

You may hear your cancer classified using the TNM Classification System. The stage of your cancer is directly related to the possibility of it spreading and causing future problems.

Tumors are designated with the letter T (tumor size), N (palpable nodes), and/or M (metastasis).

The stage of breast cancer describes its size and the extent to which it has spread. The staging system ranges from Stage I to Stage IV.

Stage	Tumor Size	Lymph Node Involvement	Metastasis (spread)
I	less than 2 cm	No	No
II	between 2–5 cm	No, or in same side	No
III	more than 5 cm	Yes, on same side	No
IV	not applicable	Not applicable	Yes

When most cancers are found, they are at the stage I or stage II levels. At these stages they are highly treatable. You doctor determines the stage by asking questions (taking a history), performing a physical examination, and doing additional tests.

Tests that help the doctor stage your cancer include a chest x-ray, bone scans, and blood tests that determine how your liver is functioning. Chest x-rays and mammograms are part of your initial assessment, and mammograms will continue to be done in the years following your treatment.

At some point in your treatment and recovery, you may undergo tests that will determine whether the disease has spread to the lungs, liver, or bone (chest x-ray, liver ultrasound, bone scan). Computerized axial tomography scans and magnetic resonance imaging scans are sometimes used if more information is needed or if the other tests don't provide enough information.

There are also good reasons for not doing these tests. They are expensive, and the chance of finding anything is relatively low. Again, remember that you have some choice in whether you want these tests. Ask your doctor what new information they might provide and how they will affect your treatment.

Should I Get a Second Opinion?

Dr. Susan Love, a U.S. surgeon and breast cancer activist, writes, "Sometimes patients are shy about seeking second opinions—as though they're somehow insulting their doctor's professionalism. Never feel that way. You're not insulting us; you're simply seeking the most precise information possible in what may literally be a life-and-death situation. Most doctors won't be offended and if you run into a doctor who does get miffed, don't be intimidated. Your life and your peace of mind are more important than your doctor's ego."

My surgeon seemed to be looking at me from a great height. He was openly angry when I sought out the cancer clinic for a second opinion.

You may want to ask your family doctor or specialist to refer you for a second opinion if you feel uncomfortable or need more information about the options being suggested to you. For women in remote and rural areas, you may have to travel to get a second opinion. Only you can determine how necessary this is for you. If you know other women who have had breast cancer, ask them who their specialists were and how they were treated. To find other breast cancer patients you can talk to, or to find out about services and support groups in your area, see the Resources section on page 142.

> "You alone know your body. You alone know when you're not feeling right. Ask questions and feel worthy. If you get unsatisfactory answers, get second, third, and fourth opinions . . . Demand answers."
>
> —JACKI RALPH JAMIESON,
> singer-songwriter

There are still many unanswered questions in the field of breast cancer research. There may not be just one answer or even a "right" answer to some of the questions you may have. Ask around. Talk to family and friends. Get as much information as you need before making any decisions.

> "Women are overwhelmed, distraught, when the diagnosis of cancer is confirmed. It is difficult at such a time to process all sorts of new and very technical facts. It is not a time when people should be pressured to make quick decisions overnight."
>
> —DR. KAREN GELMAN

There are many sources of good information. In the U.S., the National Cancer Institute's Web site is thorough and informative (see Resources section). If you are in Canada, you may find it helpful to read "Canadian Clinical Practice Guidelines for the Care and Treatment of Breast Cancer," published by the *Canadian Medical Association Journal* (CMAJ). Copies of the guidelines are available by calling the Cancer Information Service at 1-888-939-3333 or on the Web at www.cmaj.ca or www.hc-sc.gc.ca.

> *I had a very bad experience with my surgeon and hope in future women know they can ask for second opinions and not feel guilty. It was only through accident that I spoke with an oncologist and radiologist and learned that I had had an option other than the mastectomy.*

At the time of printing this book, a network of support groups for women with breast cancer is flourishing across the United States and Canada. Some individual states, regions, and provinces have their own support network as well. If you are having difficulty connecting with a support group, contact your local office of the American Cancer Society or Canadian Cancer Society.

Remember too that there are many other places to find support: among your family and friends, family doctor, nurses, and co-workers. They may be waiting for a sign from you that you want to talk—or they may be struggling to know what to do. You might want to ask a friend or family member to read this book along with you. People want to help, but you need to let them know what you need from them and when you need it.

SUMMARY

Cancer information is complex, confusing, and ever changing. You may be feeling overwhelmed with the emotional aspects of a cancer diagnosis. The information may be hard to understand. It's okay to ask questions even months or years after your diagnosis. Your doctor won't think less of you and won't consider your questions stupid or repetitive. He or she is a professional whose job is to be helpful and kind to you—not to judge you. *You* decide when you need the information.

The pathology report and other tests and scans will provide you with information that you and your doctor can use to make decisions about what to do next. Although it is only natural to assume that "more is better" when it comes to tests, you should ask your doctor to explain the tests and procedures to you so you can make an informed decision about which might be useful. It is also important to remember that some newer tests do not give any more information than the traditional markers of cancer (size, grade, hormone receptor status, and involvement of the lymph nodes) that have been used for a long time.

Staging your cancer will give you and your doctors information to plan the best treatments, help doctors communicate with each other about your case, and help to anticipate the course your disease is likely to take.

The information is based on studying many thousands of people with cancer. Although no one can predict exactly what will happen to you, it is important to understand the amount of cancer in your body to plan appropriate care.

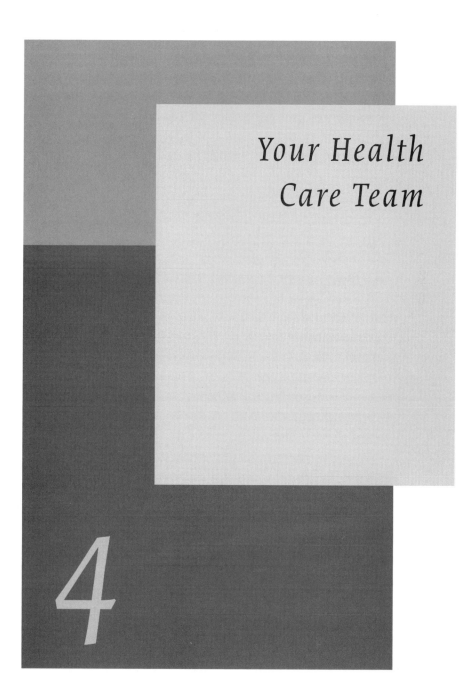

Your Health Care Team

4

This chapter is a guide to some of the people—health care professionals and others—who can help you through the diagnosis and treatment. You will also find questions that you may want to ask the people who are helping along the way.

I believe a few kind words from the doctor can go a long way.

The Other "Big C"—Communication!

Before we talk about the people who are available to help you through diagnosis and treatment, let's have a word about communication and decision-making styles. Some women are comfortable knowing very little information about their own cancer diagnosis and prefer to leave the decision making to someone else, such as a doctor they know and trust. Others want to actively participate in their diagnosis and treatment and may choose to discuss their treatment plan with family members before making any decisions. These women often feel more in control when they have this information explained to them in a way that they can understand.

No matter what your decision-making style, if you change your mind and want to talk more or less, or if you decide you want more or less information or more or less involvement in the decision making, tell your doctor. Doctors and nurses are often very good at understanding human behavior or sensing discomfort, but no one can read your mind. You'll also save yourself some time if you can make clear and understandable requests.

Try to prepare for your cancer appointments with your clinic or doctor just as you would for other important meetings. Some women may choose to ask a family member to accompany them to the appointments and help them decide what to do. Try keeping a small notebook with you to write down questions, appointment times, the name of the drugs, and the phone numbers of new people you will meet. Cancer questions or concerns can come up at any time, and some treatments cause you to become weary or forgetful. The notebook can become a useful tool or journal for your many thoughts and questions during therapy. Here are some other hints and tips:

- Let the doctor know if you want to record the meeting.
- Call ahead and ask how much time you will have for your first appointment. Let the office know if you will need a longer time or another appointment.
- Ask about directions and parking so you won't worry about them when it's time for your appointment.
- Bring along any medications, vitamins, or other treatments you are taking. Saying that you take "half a green pill and a red tablet" doesn't offer enough information.
- Tell your doctor about any other treatments or therapies such as acupuncture, herbs, vitamins, visualization, or spiritual practice that you consider important to healing.

Remember that the people who are going to care for you during cancer treatments are on your side and they know this is a very difficult time for you and your family. They are there to help you and make the treatments as understandable as possible. *You* are the most important person on your cancer-care team. *You* are the person who must make the decisions about your own care, based on the best possible advice.

Making decisions about your treatment and understanding what will happen to you may already be difficult. If you feel more comfortable speaking in a language other than English, you will probably find it helpful to bring along a friend or a family member or someone from your community who can help you.

Again, only you can determine how much information you are comfortable knowing. It will be different for each woman. If you want this information, and when you are ready to hear it, ask your doctor to write down the name of your type of breast cancer, the size of your tumor, test results, and stage of the disease.

> *I will let the doctors treat me, but the rest is up to me—whether it is mental change, cleansing teas, or exercise. Maybe by working together I will live longer or we will find a cure. I am living with cancer, not dying with cancer.*

You may have to ask more than once to be sure you understand about your treatments. Cancer information is complex and ever changing. You have the right to be given clear answers to your questions. Keep asking questions until you know everything that you want and need to know.

Who Can Help Me Get Through All This?

Your Family Doctor

Your family doctor is probably the first person you will consult. He or she will remain an important part of your cancer-care team. Family physicians rarely treat cancer, but they can and do refer you to specialists. They can be there to answer questions for you. They can play an important role in coordination, consultation, and communication. They can be your advocate in the hospital or treatment center. Ask your family doctor to refer you to a specialist in breast changes and breast cancer. Your ability to choose will depend on whether you live in or near a large urban center. If you aren't comfortable going to your appointments alone, or don't want to ask the questions yourself, ask a close friend, family member, or a woman who has been through what you are going through to help you out.

Find a family doctor you are comfortable with if you do not already have one. Some women prefer an old-fashioned, protective physician who tells them what they feel is best for them. Other women like to feel more in control and to know all about their illness. There is no right or wrong approach to this relationship. Like all long-term relationships, it is important to trust, communicate, and respect one another. This may be a lifelong relationship and requires effort by both you and your doctor.

You may also want to ask your family doctor whether you should be referred to an oncologist (cancer specialist) before surgery, if this is an option where you live. Sometimes the oncologist will consult with you and the surgeon about a treatment plan before surgery.

> *Doctors must look at the patient as a whole person. Patients must inform their physicians of what they expect from their health care providers. But God bless you if you do that. I wish people would realize that the fighters are also the survivors—they are fighting for their lives.*

Your Surgeon

In some hospitals, there are different types of surgeons, and some may specialize in breast surgery. If there is such a specialist in your hospital, this is likely whom you will see. There are some questions that you may want to ask your surgeon (or surgeons):

+ How many breast cancer patients do you treat each year?

- Do you have a preference for a certain type of surgical treatment?
- What treatment do you recommend for me and why?
- Are there advantages for me if my surgery is done at a particular time in my menstrual cycle? (If you are still menstruating)
- Can you put me in touch with a local breast cancer support group or a volunteer with Reach to Recovery?
- Can you tell me what my options are for breast reconstruction? (This does not mean you have to choose a breast reconstruction—just that you want the information.)
- Can you show me a photo of what my breast may look like after surgery?
- Can I speak with another woman you have treated?

You may want to take a husband, friend, partner, son, or daughter for support. Write down your questions and the answers. If it is difficult for you to take notes, consider taping the conversation, but let your doctor know beforehand.

Many cancer support groups have peer visitor programs for women with breast cancer. Breast cancer survivors are trained to provide support to women going through the experience of breast cancer. They can do this in the hospital, at home, or over the telephone and are matched as closely as possible by age, type of surgery, and treatment. They provide support and a free information kit, which includes booklets and other useful items.

> I found my cancer center the most caring and professional one you could wish for. One treatment nurse said to me, "You are now a cancer patient—you belong to us. We will care for you both now and after treatment and for periodic checkups afterward by your oncologist."
> These people are the greatest.

Your Oncologist

Again, depending on whether or not you live in or near a large urban center, you may be referred to an oncologist. This is the doctor whose training and experience deal specifically with cancer. Some oncologists deal with specific types of cancer, e.g., breast, brain, or lung. The two main types of oncologists are "medical oncologists" and "radiation oncologists." Medical oncologists provide systemic therapies including chemotherapy. (For more information, see Chapter 5). Radiation oncologists provide radiation treatments. Both types of treatment may be given after surgery to prevent cancer from returning.

Even if you do not have treatment after surgery, you may want to speak to an oncologist or even have your follow-up care with an oncologist. Follow-up care is the care you will need following your surgery. For some women an oncologist may not be necessary or, in certain regions of the country, available. In this case, you should see your family doctor for follow-up care.

These are some questions you or someone close to you may want to ask your oncologist or family doctor:

- What type of breast cancer do I have and at what stage is the disease?
- What treatment are you recommending for me and why?
- How will the treatment help me?
- What are the risks of the treatment?
- What can I expect to happen to me if I choose not to have this treatment?
- Will the treatments be painful? If so, how can the pain be managed?
- When and where will the treatments be?
- What are the usual side effects? Are there things you can recommend to lessen the side effects?
- How long can I expect the treatments to take?
- If I miss a treatment, can I make it up?

- What problems should I report to you?
- How can I contact you between visits?
- Can I take other medication during treatments?
- Is there anything I shouldn't eat or drink during this treatment, such as alcohol?
- What's the longest I can wait before having this treatment? (Some women want more time to fully recover from the surgery.)
- Can you put me in touch with a local breast cancer support group or a volunteer from Reach to Recovery?
- If we get rid of the cancer, what are the chances of it coming back?

Following my diagnosis and lumpectomy I felt fear every time I thought about the cancer. I bought a new car because my old one was rusting and I associated rust with cancer.

What You Can Expect from Your Health Care Team
You can expect your health care team to:

- provide information about breast cancer and treatment options
- answer your questions in a respectful and understandable way—even when you need to repeat the question several times, in different ways
- provide information about other services and resources for people with cancer in your community
- explain how to contact them between visits
- explain what kinds of symptoms you should report immediately, e.g., sudden bleeding, fever, etc.

What You Can Do to Help Your Health Care Team
Answer questions honestly. This won't be easy if you feel somewhat embarrassed, but your caregivers are there to help you, not to judge you.

If you are having problems getting the help you need, consider the following options (reprinted from the American Cancer Society).

Try working out your concerns before deciding that the situation is hopeless. First of all, state your concern as honestly and openly as possible. Here are some opening statements you may want to consider:

- "I'm concerned that we aren't communicating well, and here's why . . ."
- "I need to be able to talk with you about _____, and I feel like I can't. Can we discuss this?"
- "I realize that you're very busy, but I need very much to discuss _____ at more length. Can we schedule a time to do that?"
- "I'm having trouble understanding _____. Can you help me?"

If you need more details after your doctor answers a question, say so. Sometimes it's even helpful to ask the question again in a different way. Unless you tell your doctor that you don't understand something, he or she will usually assume that you do. There's nothing wrong with not understanding the first explanation; just ask for another.

If you want to learn more about your cancer treatment, ask your doctor to suggest some reading materials. If you feel comfortable doing so, learning more about your treatment can also help you become more actively involved in it.

If you are unable to work out the problem during your regular visits with your doctor, ask for a special visit to discuss it. If the issue directly concerns your cancer treatment, go to the meeting with as much knowledge as possible. Always tell your doctor where you get your information and then ask for his or her opinion.

Even if you feel frustrated or angry, try to avoid being hostile or accusatory toward your doctor. Much of the time, people will become defensive and withdrawn if they feel attacked—a response that will be unhelpful in the long run. State your concerns and questions clearly and honestly, without making accusations.

What should you do if you feel you have done your part but the situation has not improved? You might consider talking with a third party about the problem. The head nurse or your family doctor might be willing to discuss the matter with the doctor. Sometimes this is less stressful than facing the doctor directly, and their help could improve the situation. If not, it may be time to find a new doctor. Don't stay with a doctor only to protect his or her feelings. Just because you were referred to the doctor does not mean you can't decide to change on your own. It's your body and you have the right to find the best doctor for you.

COUNSELORS

Doctors and surgeons are trained to deal with cancer tumors, but you are also learning to live with the confusion and pain that follows a diagnosis of cancer. To help you cope with the emotional and spiritual side of cancer, you may want to talk to a counselor experienced in the particular problems and challenges cancer brings to our lives. Some cities now even have therapists who specialize in counseling cancer patients and families. The people whom you love, particularly your partner, your children, other family members, and friends, also need emotional support to help you and to cope with their own fear.

> I still feel the need to talk to survivors but never make the contact because in our city, I would have to initiate such a support group, and I don't have a lot of energy emotionally. If there was such a group I would join. At times I want to forget about the cancer and pretend it never happened, but it haunts me day and night. I want to deal with the anger and fear in a safe place.

Cancer Survivors

It may be helpful and comforting to be able to talk to a woman who, like you, has learned to live with cancer. If you do not already know such a woman, check the Resources section on page 142 for support groups in your area. Some women have found it helpful to get in touch with such a group or individual before they have any surgery or treatment. The women involved with these groups have had breast cancer and have found their strength again. They will be able to share their experience with you, and many are gentle, informed listeners.

> *I am extremely happy and satisfied with my treatment at the cancer center. The one thing missing, however, was any information about support groups. Even now, after four years, I still feel the need to talk to someone other than my family and friends about my cancer.*

Other Sources of Support

Nurses, social workers, psychologists, and other types of health care providers can often be helpful to people who are fighting cancer. They may be able to answer your questions about treatment and how you can expect to feel; they can also help you work through the emotional and spiritual issues that may arise from facing cancer. You may be able to find this kind of help by talking with friends or family, asking at your cancer treatment center, or contacting your local breast cancer support group.

A nurse, counselor, social worker, or friend may be able to help you as you work through some of these questions either before or after your surgery:

- What can I do to rebuild my health?
- How will I look after surgery? Will I need a breast prosthesis? How can I decide if I want breast reconstruction?

- Can you show me a picture of what it would look like afterward? (Some women show each other their mastectomy or lumpectomy scars in support groups.)
- How might this affect me sexually?
- What might people say and how will I answer? How might I deal with their concern or their pity?
- How can I deal with the pain?
- What have I learned from the experts I've seen and what is going to work for me, for my life, and for my survival?
- I feel badly about not taking care of my partner, my family, my friends, my job. What can I do?

Friends, family, members of your cultural community, and, possibly, clergy can also help with their love and support. Take what you learn from these people and use it to take charge of your survival!

I was fortunate to have good friends rally round me, not just in the beginning but throughout. To the ones who left, I can honestly say a gentle good-bye.

SUMMARY

You are the most important person on your cancer-care team. You are the one who must design your own treatment plan based on what you learn about your disease and from talking to others. Surround yourself with whomever you need to support yourself through this time, including other women who have been through what you are going through.

I'm learning to live with fear—and reach for support. I watch a lot more sunsets and do a lot less homework.

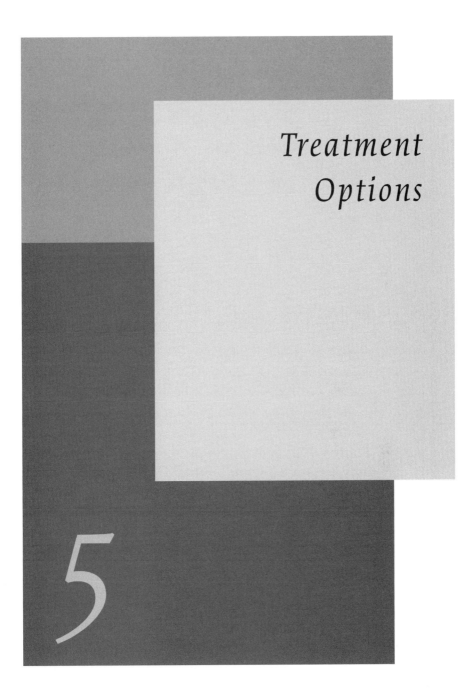

Treatment
Options

5

This chapter will discuss the next steps in helping you to understand and choose your treatment option.

> "Tomorrow will be 'look at my bare chest' day. I have been protected by bandages for a week. Now I must face the fact. I have but one breast. And a scar. Some champagne perhaps? To celebrate the new image."
>
> —BARB SULLIVAN,
> *My Broken Breast Book*

How Do I Choose?

There are many different approaches to the treatment of breast cancer, including surgery, with or without radiation, often in combination with chemotherapy and other drug treatments. This chapter will explain what some of the many treatments are, when they are appropriate, and how to weigh the risks and benefits of each choice. These decisions will be based upon the information you already have about your type of cancer, the pathology report, your age, other health factors, and your preferences (see the chart on page 91 for some options).

Again, one important source of information is the "Canadian Clinical Practice Guidelines for the Care and Treatment of Breast Cancer" published by the *Canadian Medical Association Journal* (CMAJ). To receive a copy, contact the Cancer Information Service at 1-888-939-3333 or on the Web at www.cmaj.ca. or www.hc-sc.gc.ca. In the U.S., visit the National Cancer Institute Web site at www.nci.nih.gov.

The information contained in this chapter is targeted to women who have already had a biopsy, know they have breast cancer, and are now considering what to do next. Once you have been diagnosed, there are a number of decisions concerning which treatment or combination of treatments will offer you the best possibility of a long and healthy survival. Remember, there is no single right treatment for everyone. Your breast cancer treatment choices will depend on many factors.

You may want to take a friend or a family member along for support when you discuss treatments. Remember to write down your questions and the answers. If it is difficult for you to take notes, you may want to consider taping the conversation. If so, let your doctor know you would like to do so beforehand.

> Canada and the United States offer some of the best cancer treatment in the world. But in an increasingly complex medical system, women must be aggressive, skeptical, sharp, and savvy consumers to make sure they get it. At the very moment when they see their lives falling apart, when mortality looms large, they must turn themselves into shrewd shoppers.

Treatment Options

Treatments for breast cancer are generally divided into two categories: local treatment of the breast or lymph gland regions, such as surgery and radiation, and systemic treatment for the rest of the body, such as chemotherapy and/or hormone therapy. In addition, there are some unconventional therapies that some people choose to complement traditional cancer therapy.

LOCAL TREATMENTS: SURGERY
Almost all women with breast cancer will have some type of surgery (see Figure 5.1). The type of surgery will depend on a number of things that you should discuss with your surgeon. You will probably have

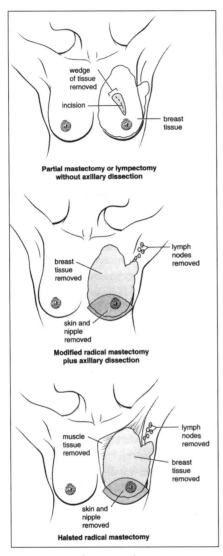

wedge
of tissue
removed

incision

breast
tissue

**Partial mastectomy or lympectomy
without axillary dissection**

lymph
nodes
removed

breast
tissue
removed

skin and
nipple
removed

**Modified radical mastectomy
plus axillary dissection**

lymph
nodes
removed

muscle
tissue
removed

breast
tissue
removed

skin and
nipple
removed

Halsted radical mastectomy

FIGURE 5.1   *Three types of surgery*

your initial surgery at a local hospital, depending on where your surgeon works. Usually the most convenient choice is the center closest to home.

The surgeon saw me on Thursday and advised an immediate mastectomy, which I had the following day. He was kindness personified and I was sure he was right. I felt a tremendous sense of urgency to "get on" with my surgery. Looking back on the good and bad aspects of my personal experience, being advised to have immediate surgery was good, but I wish I had taken more time to consider my options.

Simple Mastectomy

Simple mastectomy surgery will include the removal of all the breast tissue that normally fits into your bra. The surgeon does not remove any of the underlying chest muscles—the pectoralis major or the pectoralis minor. The lymphatic tissue in your armpit and shoulder area is also not removed.

Modified Radical Mastectomy

Modified radical mastectomy removes the breast and lymph nodes and leaves the chest muscles intact. Modified radical mastectomy has proven as effective as the more radical surgery.

Mastectomy is a good choice for women who:

+ are not able to have radiation treatment after lumpectomy
+ have large tumors or multiple sites of tumors in a small breast
+ have a high risk of recurrence in the same breast
+ have a personal preference for mastectomy

The Halstead radical mastectomy is the removal of the entire breast, chest wall muscles beneath the breast, and some of the underarm or axillary lymph nodes. This surgery is no longer performed.

> *I went into the hospital in 1946 for what the doctors thought was a small benign lump but which turned out to be a malignant tumor. I had a child a year and a half later and have been married to a wonderful man for fifty years. I think that things have come a long way since. I do not regret that a complete radical was done as I have never worried about it since. They also did not give you many choices in the Good Old Days.*

Partial Mastectomy/Lumpectomy

The alternative to a modified radical mastectomy is a surgery that removes only the cancerous section and a margin of the surrounding normal breast tissue. Partial mastectomy, lumpectomy, breast-conserving surgery, wide excision, segmental mastectomy, and quadrantectomy are all names you may hear used for this operation. The part removed can be anywhere from 1 percent to 25 percent of the breast tissue. Standard treatment following a partial mastectomy or lumpectomy is radiation treatment (Figures 5.2 and 5.3). In almost all cases, four to six weeks of radiation therapy will follow surgery.

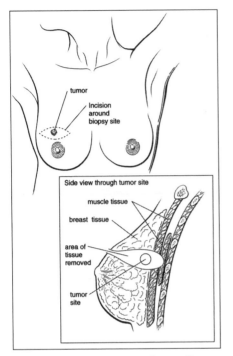

Inside the figure:
tumor
Incision
around
biopsy site

Side view through tumor site
muscle tissue
breast tissue
area of
tissue
removed
tumor
site

FIGURE 5.2 *Lumpectomy without axillary dissection (no lymph nodes removed)*

There are some women who should not have a lumpectomy:

- women who have had previous radiation treatment to the chest or breast
- women with two or more areas of cancer in the same breast
- women with connective tissue disorders (e.g., lupus erythematosis) that make them sensitive to radiation and may prevent them from healing
- pregnant women

For women who have a lumpectomy, it is important to know if the margins (edges) of the lumpectomy specimen are "clear" or free of cancer. Sometimes the surgeon won't know this until the specimen has been examined by a pathologist. The surgeon generally takes a wide margin around the tumor; nonetheless, he or she cannot see what is going on at the cellular level.

Women should ask the surgeon if the tumor margins were clear. Sometimes patients arrive to see their oncologist assuming that the tumor was clear, only to find out that more surgery or an extra "boost" of radiation to the tumor bed may be needed.

Axillary Lymph Node Dissection or Sentinel Node Biopsy

The surgeon may also remove fat and lymph nodes from the armpit area to find out if there are any cancer cells spreading beyond the breast tissue. The lymph nodes are part of the system that carries fluid, called "lymph," around the body. When breast cancer spreads, it often collects in the lymph nodes in the armpit area. By surgically removing the nodes and examining them under a microscope, the pathologist can determine if the nodes are "positive" (containing cancer cells) or "negative" (no cancer cells).

Rather than removing all or most of the underarm lymph nodes, a "sentinel node" biopsy may be considered. During a sentinel node biopsy, radioactive material or a dye (or both) is injected into the breast tissue surrounding the tumor. As the lymph carries the dye through the lymphatic pathways, the surgeon uses a device that identifies whether the first lymph node—the sentinel node—is free of cancer. If it is, then no other lymph nodes need to be removed and the surgery has minimal side effects. The sentinel lymph node is thought to accurately reflect the state of all of the nodes in the armpit. There is always a small chance (in some cases as high as 10 percent) that even though no cancer cells are found in the sentinel node, some cancer cells still lurk in other nodes; this can affect the success of treatments. If the sentinel node is positive for cancer, than an axillary dissection should be performed.

What Will Surgery Be Like?

Depending on the type of surgery you have and how soon you recover, your hospital stay may last only one or two days. The length of your stay may also depend on the region of the country you live in. You are usually asked to check into the hospital early the same day as your surgery. The anesthesiologist will likely visit you briefly and should answer any questions you may ask. Let him or her know if you have had problems such as nausea, vomiting, severe or unusual pain, or other side effects with previous surgery and recovery. Be sure to tell the anesthesiologist if a close blood relative has had any difficulties with an anesthetic. You will not be allowed to eat or drink from the evening before the surgery until after you have been brought back from the recovery room.

Depending on the type, the surgery will likely take from two to four hours. Following surgery, your breast will be bandaged and one or two tubes will be in place to drain fluid from the wound. Your throat may be sore from the airway tube that was in place during surgery. You may feel sick to your stomach and tired. There may be numbness, tingling, or pain in your chest, shoulder, or arm. Some women feel pain in the breast they have lost. If you are in pain, you can ask for medication. It is important for you to rest after the surgery and regain your strength.

Among the possible short-term side effects of both mastectomy and lumpectomy are the following:

+ wound infection
+ hematoma or blood that accumulates in the wound
+ seroma or accumulation of clear fluid in the wound, which can be drained

Long-term effects may include:

+ pain or "postmastectomy syndrome" that is caused by nerve damage
+ lymphedema or swelling caused by removal of the lymph glands, which can happen even years after surgery

Medication can help manage the pain rapidly and completely. Compression and massage can help manage chronic pain from lymphedema. And there are alternative therapies such as meditation, biofeedback, yoga, prayer, visualization, Tai Chi, therapeutic touch, and herbal remedies. Although there is not sufficient scientific evidence about these therapies, many patients report significant benefits.

Pain can also be caused by the emotional distress of a cancer diagnosis and can be made worse because of fear, depression, or anxiety. Talking to friends, family, support group members, or professional counselors can help you to manage this difficult time.

Shortly after surgery, when you have had some time to rest, your surgeon will probably meet with you to discuss the surgery. He or she may comment on the amount of tissue removed and the number of lymph nodes sent to the lab for biopsy. The results of the lymph node biopsy will help determine the stage of your disease.

Before Leaving the Hospital

This is often a very difficult time as you wait for the lab reports. The amount of time it will take for the lab results to come back can vary greatly from one hospital to another and one region to the next. Some women have found this a particularly difficult time, as you may wait wondering and worrying about the future, imagining all kinds of things happening to you. You may find it helpful to talk to your nurses and caregivers about your feelings. You may want to talk with someone from your local breast cancer support group, if there is one in your area. They can arrange a hospital or home visit, organize a group meeting, or provide support by telephone.

> *The time it took for the diagnosis to be available after the lumpectomy was especially long—almost one week. It was the longest week in my life. Maybe my case was exceptional, but anything done to speed up the time would have been appreciated.*

Before you leave the hospital, you should be shown how to care for your surgical wound. Ask when it is all right to shave or use deodorant (most deodorants contain aluminum, which may interfere with radiation treatments). Ask when the stitches will be removed. The stitches are usually removed a week later by either your family doctor or your surgeon. Many surgeons use dissolving stitches, which don't need to be removed. It may be two to four weeks before you feel ready to drive or go back to work. Some women have found that shoulder-strap car seat belts are irritating if they rub against the scar. You may want to put a soft cloth between the belt and you.

For a few weeks or more, you may want to wear soft, loose-fitting clothing as the scar heals. If your surgery was a mastectomy, when the scar has healed you may choose to wear a soft breast, called a "prosthesis," in your bra. Temporary prostheses are often available free of charge from a Reach to Recovery volunteer or from your local support group. If you are not having further treatment (radiation or chemotherapy), you may be able to have breast reconstruction surgery at the same time as your mastectomy or soon after, if you wish. It is wise to discuss this option with your surgeon during your visits before surgery.

Like many women, you may feel comfortable with your changed body just as it is and not choose breast reconstruction. Some women simply don't want to go through any more surgery. There are a number of possible options you may want to consider. You may need to take some time (and this may be months or years) to become fully comfortable in choosing the right option for you.

Keeping Active

Whether you had a mastectomy or a lumpectomy, if lymph nodes were removed, your arm may be weak. If it is not routinely offered in your hospital, you may request to meet with someone from the rehabilitation or physiotherapy department who is knowledgeable about breast cancer to learn exercises that will help regain the strength in your arm and maintain mobility. These exercises are an important part of your recovery and will prevent muscles in the arm and shoulder from becoming "frozen" or stiff. Whether you get help with exercising in the hospital or plan your own exercises, keep active in order to prevent long-term problems with circulation and movement.

Lymphedema

Some women develop a condition called "lymphedema," which is a swelling in the arm or hand because the lymph nodes are not properly draining the lymph fluid. Although it is becoming less common as surgical techniques become more sophisticated, lymphedema can happen any time after the surgery (even years later) and it may be temporary or permanent.

My only regret is lymphedema in my arm. I wish I could get relief from this. It is very annoying during short-sleeve season. Otherwise I am happy to have had the surgery and I've been healthy ever since. This is all I have to bear.

If lymphedema (Figure 5.3) develops, a compression sleeve for the arm can be helpful. Some women have also found massage therapy to be helpful for arm problems after surgery. Therapeutic massage by a registered massage therapist (RMT) can help to increase blood flow and lymph flow at a time when it will be difficult for you to enjoy these benefits from exercise. Some people have expressed concerns that stimulating blood and lymph flow might activate cancer cells or cause them to spread. No research has demonstrated this to be so. If you are going to have massage therapy, you may want to discuss this issue with both your physician and your massage therapist. Most certified massage therapists are qualified to do both "deep-tissue" massage and a lighter approach that may help you to relax and improve circulation. If you are at all concerned about the possible discomfort from deep-tissue massage, you may want to request a light massage therapy approach.

Many women experience numbness and a change in feeling around their scar, which sometimes travels through the arm. This is caused by the nerves that have been cut during surgery and are healing. The numbness may diminish in a year or so, but in some women it may last longer. You may find it helpful to use a small soft pillow to support the arm when you are sitting or lying down. The changed feeling around the surgery site may not always be unpleasant. Some women have reported the feeling as pleasant, even sensual.

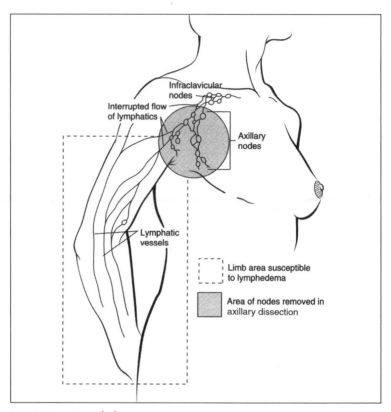

FIGURE 5.3 *Lymphedema*

LOCAL TREATMENTS: RADIATION THERAPY

A partial mastectomy or lumpectomy is usually followed by radiation treatment to the breast (see Figures 5.4 and 5.5). Radiation treatment helps prevent a recurrence of cancer in the breast. Although many specialists consider this treatment standard and necessary after surgery, it is important to remember that you have a choice in this. If your tumor was very small, less than .05 cm, and non-invasive, and you had a lumpectomy, you may be able to avoid radiation. You should discuss this with your oncologist. However, radiation is still considered standard for small tumors.

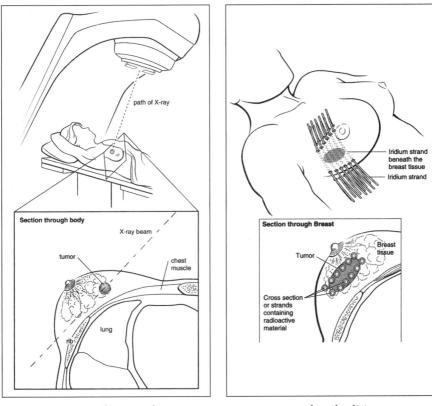

FIGURE 5.4 *How radiation works*   FIGURE 5.5 *Implanted radioisotopes*

The chance of recurrence is greater in younger women (under age forty-six) than older women (over seventy), so this factor should be considered, as well.

Radiation therapy takes place five days a week for four to six weeks. Radiation treatment uses high-energy x-rays to kill cancer cells and shrink tumors by heating the cells to a high temperature. The radiation can also cause "sunburn" and red, sore skin.

External radiation is done by machines that direct the x-rays to precise areas of the body, such as a part of the breast. This is the type of radiation that most women receive. A smaller number of women receive internal radiation therapy, which involves implanting thin plastic tubes into the breast area at the site of your tumor. The tubes contain materials that produce radiation (radioisotopes). This method of treatment has not been evaluated in randomized trials, and for the time being, the results cannot be considered equal to external radiation.

Radiation treatments affect only the area to which the x-rays are directed. Marks will be put on your breast and you will be asked not to wash them off until treatment is complete. Sometimes the marks are tattooed, becoming permanent.

Because radiation therapy treatments require the use of sophisticated and expensive machinery, they are usually available only in specialized cancer centers and certain hospitals. This may require that you travel on a daily basis or stay away from home for a period of four to six weeks. Many cancer centers make arrangements to assist patients with daily travel (volunteer drivers) or staying overnight (such as lodge accommodations). Ask the staff at the treatment center if you can take advantage of this assistance.

For women who have the following health conditions, radiation therapy is not a good choice:

- pregnancy
- previous radiation treatment to the breast or chest area
- arthritis that prevents you from lying flat for a long period with arms extended
- systemic lupus erythematosus
- scleroderma

Systemic Adjuvant Treatments

If after surgery your lymph nodes show that the cancer has spread, or if the lymph nodes are negative for cancer but there are other worrisome features, your doctor should discuss systemic treatments with you.

Systemic treatment is used to treat cancer throughout the body, in every cell. Ask questions and consider getting the opinion of a medical oncologist if further treatment is recommended for you.

Systemic treatments are used to treat cancer cells that may have traveled from the breast tumor to other parts of the body through the blood system or the lymph system. There are two types of systemic therapy: chemotherapy and hormone therapy. Sometimes they are used separately, sometimes they are combined. Hormone therapy is used only with estrogen receptor positive tumors. When very small cancer cells have been found in the lymph nodes, there is a chance that the cancer may also have spread to other parts of the body. Be sure to ask your cancer specialist to describe why chemotherapy is being recommended if there are no cancer cells in the lymph nodes.

For large tumors, chemotherapy or radiation is sometimes given before surgery to shrink the size (this is called neo-adjuvant treatment). In this case, you might be referred to an oncologist before surgery, or you might ask for a referral before deciding on treatment.

Chemotherapy

Chemotherapy uses drugs, taken by injection or in pill form, to kill cancer cells (Figure 5.6). The drugs work by preventing the cells from dividing or reproducing, which forces them to die. But the drugs are not very selective. They may kill other healthy cells that are also dividing, including hair cells and bone marrow cells. This explains why some women lose their hair during chemotherapy treatments. In the bone marrow, the drugs lower the body's production of red and white blood cells and platelets. This can affect your energy level, your ability to fight off infection, and the ability of your blood to clot properly. Remember that these effects are only temporary. Your blood cells will begin to function normally once you have stopped having treatments.

Adjuvant Breast Cancer Treatment Options for Patients

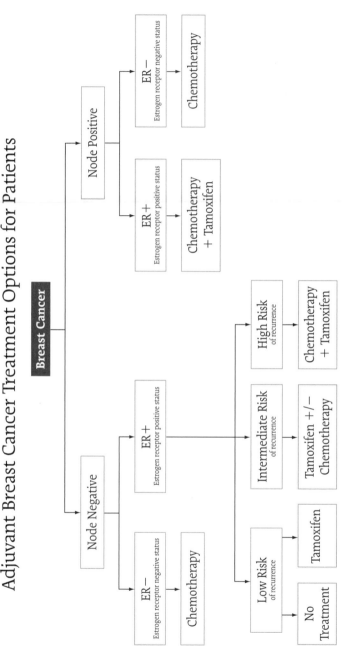

Adapted from: Abraham eds., et al. *Bethesda Handbook of Clinical Oncology.* Lippincott, Williams & Wilkins, 2001, 131, and from the Canadian Guidelines for node negative and node positive breast cancer in the CMAJ.

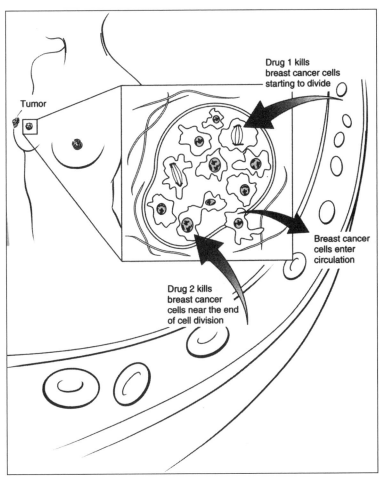

Drug 1 kills
breast cancer cells
starting to divide

Tumor

Breast cancer
cells enter
circulation

Drug 2 kills
breast cancer
cells near the end
of cell division

FIGURE 5.6 *Chemotherapy combines several drugs that act on breast cancer cells at different stages of cell division.*

Research has shown that chemotherapy drugs are more effective when used in combination rather than singly. The most frequently used combinations are:

- Cyclophosphamide, methotrexate, and fluorouracil (CMF)
- Cyclophosphamide, epirubicin, and fluorouracil (CEF)

- Doxorubicin (Adriamycin) and cyclophosphamide (AC), with or without paclitaxel (Taxol) (ACT). Preliminary results of a recent study in women with early breast cancer show that the combination of taxotere, doxorubicin, and cyclophosphamide (TAC) is very promising. It is a reasonable treatment option to discuss with your doctor.

The drugs are given in weekly cycles lasting three to four weeks (depending on the regimen), with each period of treatment followed by a period of recovery. The duration of treatment is usually between three and six months. Ask your oncologist to explain your particular chemotherapy treatment to you. The side effects will depend on the type of drugs used, the length of treatment, and the amount taken.

Chemotherapy is usually given following the initial surgery. Radiation is usually given after the chemotherapy is completed. Chemotherapy treatments are usually given in specialized cancer treatment centers but can also be administered through community clinics or hospital outpatient departments. The location will depend on where you live and which oncologist you see. Be sure to advise your dentist, chiropractor, or other health care providers that you are in chemotherapy treatment. A dental checkup before starting chemotherapy may be helpful to avoid any bleeding problems caused by the drugs.

Hormone Therapy

Medications such as tamoxifen (Nolvadex) interfere with your body's hormones to lessen the growth of certain estrogen-sensitive tumors. The side effects of these drugs may not be as harsh as chemotherapy, but their purpose is the same: to keep cancer cells from growing. Tamoxifen works by blocking the uptake of estrogen by the cancer cells.

A lot of media attention has been given to tamoxifen in the past few years. Most of the controversy has to do with using tamoxifen to try to prevent breast cancer in healthy women. Researchers have found a link to the development of uterine cancer in humans and liver cancer in animals. But what is a risk for well women is not the same level of risk for a woman who already has breast cancer and uses the drug as treatment, not prevention.

If your doctor is recommending tamoxifen for you, ask about side effects such as vaginal spotting or bleeding, blood clots, or changes in your vision.

Aromatase Inhibitors   Early findings about a new class of hormone-modifying drugs, called aromatase inhibitors, show that they may be better than tamoxifen in preventing recurrence of breast cancer. They include anastrozole (Arimidex), letrozole (Femara), and exemestane (Aromasin). These drugs have been used for several years to treat advanced disease or metastatic breast cancer. Unlike tamoxifen, which counteracts the effects of estrogen and has side effects such as possible endometrial cancer, blood clots, and cataracts, aromatase inhibitors interfere with the production of estrogen. Aromatase inhibitors don't help strengthen bones and can cause menopausal symptoms, so they are not recommended for women who are premenopausal.

OOPHORECTOMY

A less common treatment for estrogen receptor positive breast cancer patients nowadays is the removal of the ovaries, or oophorectomy, which removes the woman's primary source of estrogen. This treatment was common before the development of anti-estrogen drugs, like tamoxifen, and is still occasionally recommended for women who are premenopausal. Ovarian ablation can also be achieved with a medication called Zoludex. Zoludex interferes with the pituitary gland's ability to stimulate the ovaries' production of estrogen.

UNCONVENTIONAL THERAPIES

More and more people in North America are looking to unconventional therapies not only to prevent illness but also to help them recover from illness. Many of these therapies have not been put through rigorous scientific testing to prove whether or not they are effective. Also, as many cancer patients have learned, medical doctors sometimes view them as "quackery." It is important to remember, however, that many of the treatments we have come to view as standard cancer care (such as radiation) were also once viewed as "quackery" and dismissed by the medical profession. Some medical doctors view any unconventional therapies as useless because their effectiveness has not been scientifically proven.

"Modern medicine has largely focused on the physical side of the problem, aggressively attacking the illness, often ignoring the person who has it. On the other hand, 'alternative medicine' has focused on the person rather than the disease, insisting that it is simply 'mind over matter': fix it in your mind and the physical problem will take care of itself. This approach is equally wrong. It is the interaction of the mind and body that matters. Coping with illness is both a mental and physical process."

—DR. DAVID SPIEGEL,
Living beyond Limits: New Hope and
Help for Facing Life-Threatening Illness

There was a time when the foods we ate were not seen to play a role in the development of cancer. We now know from research that certain types of food eaten on a regular basis—like broccoli, cauliflower, and brussels sprouts—can help prevent the development of certain types of cancer. As well, some unconventional therapies gaining popularity in Western countries today have been used for centuries in other cultures and countries, such as herbal remedies and acupuncture. The health care community's understanding of which unconventional treatments work and which don't is continually evolving.

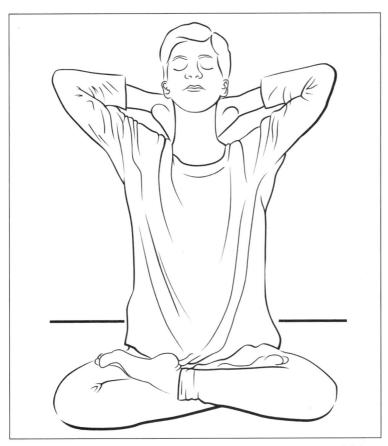

FIGURE 5.7   *Self-healing techniques focus on the mind-body connection and directing the body's own spiritual energy toward healing.*

We sometimes refer to unconventional therapies as "complementary" because they may be used alongside standard medical treatments to improve the chance of recovery. Some treatments, such as vitamin therapy, could help to strengthen your body's natural ability to fight disease. But it is important not to abandon potentially helpful conventional therapies if you plan to also explore unconventional ones.

"It's heartbreaking when women die of breast cancer because they were too scared to take chemotherapy and radiation. As in my case, these aggressive treatments were highly successful against breast cancer. There is a complementary role, however, for alternative therapies to help us regain and maintain our well-being—and to help prevent illness in the first place. But it is very confusing for people to distinguish what is useful when conventional practitioners are unwilling to consider anything that doesn't come from pharmaceutical companies. I've found value in many dietary, herbal, and vitamin supports, and in exercise, visualization, and progressive relaxation. More openness about complementary aids might help people to not chase the rainbow of 'miracle cures' that do no more than drain financial resources, while also increasing individual responsibility for our health."

—ANNE SWARBRICK,
breast cancer survivor, former Member
of the Ontario Provincial Parliament

Our mental and spiritual states are linked in very important ways to the physical workings of our bodies. There is a belief that the mind can help to heal the body and promote well-being. Techniques that focus on the mind-body connection include meditation, prayer, relaxation techniques, laughter therapy, and visualization. These techniques can reduce the pain and uncomfortable side effects of treatment by stimulating the production of endorphins, which are natural painkillers produced in the brain. For some people, prayer and other spiritual practices have similar effects.

One of the difficulties that cancer patients face is finding reliable information about unconventional therapies and someone who can help them sort out what they need. Some states and provinces have legislation that governs health care providers who work with certain unconventional therapies. These include naturopaths, acupuncturists, herbalists, massage therapists, chiropractors, and osteopaths. Often you can find out more about unconventional therapies and health care providers who are knowledgeable about them in breast cancer support groups.

If you are interested in pursuing unconventional therapies as part of your cancer treatment, first gather as much information as you can. Then talk about it with your health care team. Patients should not be afraid to discuss alternative therapies with their doctors. There needs to be mutual understanding and respect, and if the patient chooses complementary or alternative therapies, this should not prejudice care. However, if the doctor is not keen, the patient should respect the doctor's values.

It is still not fully known which of the available complementary therapies can help you physically, but some can certainly help you in a spiritual and emotional sense. It is important for you to keep in mind that only you can decide what is right for you. Healing is what your body does for itself. Affirming the love and support that is available from family, friends, and our own selves can reduce the helplessness and loneliness brought on by a cancer diagnosis.

Clinical Trials

You may be interested in joining clinical trials of new treatments. Clinical trials are designed by scientists, and approved in the U.S. by the Food and Drug Administration (FDA) and in Canada by the Therapeutics Program Directorate of Health Canada, to study and compare new treatments with those that have already been proven effective and are available. It was through clinical trials that many of today's standard treatments were proven effective. A new drug must go through three phases of clinical trials before it is approved by a regulatory agency.

Phase I   This stage of development focuses on the safety and side effects, the best way to administer the drug, and how much to give. Doctors pay careful attention to side effects and patients are carefully monitored. Drugs in phase I studies have already been proven to be safe in laboratory studies with animals, but the effects on people are not yet well understood.

Phase II   After the drug's safety has been determined, its effectiveness can be evaluated. Patients are very carefully monitored to determine the drug's effect on the cancer; for example, does it shrink in size. Baseline studies will be done before you start treatment to measure any changes. Again, the side effects are carefully assessed.

Phase III   These are often very large studies with hundreds of participants. There will be a "control group" of patients who receive the standard treatment, and another group of patients who receive the "study" or experimental treatment. In this way, researchers can compare the two treatments to find out what differences occur. The decision as to which patients receive the experimental drug and which receive the standard treatment is made by random allocation (like flipping a coin) by a computer. Again, participants are carefully monitored for side effects and studies can be discontinued if the side effects are severe.

Participating in clinical trials is voluntary, which will be very carefully explained to you and your family. Detailed explanations about the clinical trial will be provided in a written format, along with informed consent documents. The informed consent documents state that you understand the clinical trial and the potential risks; if you agree to participate in the trial, you must sign the consent forms. Clinical trials are approved by your cancer center or hospital's research ethics board.

You can leave the study at any time and for any reason. Participating in clinical trials can be an appropriate choice at any stage in your treatment. Although the trial may or may not benefit you directly, clinical trials are the best hope for improving future outcomes for breast cancer patients. You will be carefully monitored and your care and treatment will be as good as (and possibly better than) standard treatments.

SUMMARY

After breast cancer has been confirmed by biopsy, other treatments will follow—likely including some kind of surgery. Radiation may follow the surgery. If there is evidence of disease in the lymph nodes or elsewhere, or if the tumor looks large or aggressive, you will likely have a form of systemic drug treatment—either chemotherapy or hormone therapy or both. If you receive chemotherapy, radiation will be administered after completion. Participating in a clinical trial for new treatments is a consideration for all patients.

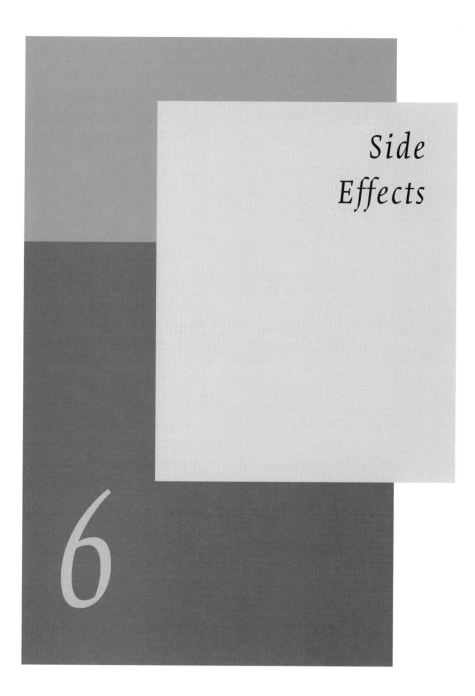

Side
Effects

6

This chapter discusses some of the common effects of treatment. Most cancer treatments do have some side effects, and these can cause stress. Knowing what to anticipate can help you cope and reduce anxiety. Remember that everybody reacts differently. You may have all, some, or none of the side effects discussed here.

One year of chemo left me tired and feeling "icky"—but I still carried on my regular life most of the time.

What Side Effects Can I Expect from the Surgery and Treatments?

Most cancer treatments will have some side effects, and they all create stress. Stress can make you irritable, tired, and depressed. Anesthesia, surgery, chemotherapy, and radiation are also frightening. They, too, can cause depression and tiredness. Other side effects after surgery may include infection, tenderness, pain, scarring, lymphedema, and possibly reduced movement if you do not regularly exercise the affected arm. To prevent infection of the skin of the arm, chest, or breast (called cellulitis), it is important to avoid cuts, scrapes, bruises, or infection in the hand and arm after surgery and/or radiation.

Before my operation I was frightened and felt alone, confused, and too depressed to seek advice. The pamphlets described medical procedures adequately but didn't begin to tell me about all the little troubles I would have to face after the operation, such as the pain and how to ease it without overmedicating, how to get a coat on, the most beneficial arm exercises, the discomfort of radiation burns. I found the best solution was to wrap the burned area in an old soft sweatshirt. A book of practical tips would be appreciated by a lot of women, I'm sure.

Try to get as much rest as possible, exercise moderately, and eat as well as you can. Looking after yourself can help you cope with treatment.

Following my mastectomy, I couldn't use my arm for a few months, and lived with pain for more than a year. Since then, everything has gone back to normal.

CHEMOTHERAPY SIDE EFFECTS

Reactions to chemotherapy will vary depending on the individual and which drugs are used. Some of the frequent side effects are tiredness, weakness, body aches, bloating and weight gain, changes in your complexion, night sweats, nausea or vomiting, and changes in your sense of taste and smell. If you are experiencing nausea or vomiting, ask your health care provider for anti-nausea medication. Some antinausea drugs work better than others. Keep trying until you find one that works for you.

My life was measured by chemo days. One week of the month I was guaranteed to be ill. It would take two weeks to recover and finally one week of feeling well before it all began again. I thank God for my family and friends, who helped me through this trip to hell. With my chemo days behind me, I can show all the people in my life how much I truly love them.

Infection

Sometimes, chemotherapy will lower your white blood cell count, making you more prone to an infection such as pneumonia. If you run a temperature of more than 38.5°C while on chemotherapy you should call your health care team immediately. (If you don't have a thermometer, it would be a good idea to get one.) If you do get an infection, it has likely come from bacteria that normally live in harmony on or in your body. Infections are rarely "caught" from someone else. You don't need to live in a "glass bubble;" just use good common sense.

Forgetfulness and Mood Swings (a.k.a. "Chemo-brain")

Women have also commented that chemotherapy seemed to make them feel depressed and forgetful, or cause dramatic mood swings. These changes are temporary, but they can last as long as two years after finishing chemotherapy. It might help to talk with a friend, family member, counselor, or another woman living with breast cancer. The moods that accompany cancer treatment are a common topic at support groups, and it might help you to manage these side effects if you can talk to another patient.

Changes in Menstrual Cycle

If you menstruate, your periods will likely become irregular or may stop altogether. For many women, their periods return when treatment is over. For some who have not yet gone through menopause, chemotherapy can cause the ovaries to stop producing estrogen and lead to an earlier menopause.

Mouth Sores

Some people develop mouth sores during chemotherapy. Rinse your mouth with a solution of baking soda and water often during the day to clean and refresh your mouth. Drink eight to ten glasses of water and choose foods that are easy to swallow. For this side effect, and others such as diarrhea, you may want to speak to a nutritionist or members of a support group.

Taste Changes

Many people find that food doesn't taste the same during treatments. Meat especially may have a bitter or metallic taste. Choosing chicken, turkey, or fish, and using plastic utensils can help. Also limit caffeine intake.

Hygiene

Women have found it helpful to pay extra attention to hygiene and allow themselves plenty of time to rest and recuperate to decrease the chances of additional sickness or infection.

Hair Loss

One of the greatest fears about chemotherapy is losing your hair. But hair does grow back after treatment ends. Also, women generally don't lose the hair under their arms or in the pubic area. Whether or not hair loss occurs depends on the particular drugs you will be receiving. Some drugs never cause hair loss while others always do. Others have different effects on the hair. Some women believe that losing hair will strip away their femininity. Hair loss may feel like a very public statement that they have cancer. If you are going to lose your hair, it may become thin or you may lose it suddenly. It may come out in clumps. Frequently it will happen about three to four weeks after your first treatment.

Some women choose to wear scarves or turbans; others buy wigs. It is important to be fitted for your wig so that it looks good on you and doesn't fall off. Don't send someone else out to buy it. If possible, choose a wig ahead of time so that the fitter can see what you look like with hair, or bring a picture of yourself to the fitting. Some women have their hair cut very short just before starting chemotherapy. If you do this, keep some of your hair for fitters to use as bangs for a turban. This sometimes helps women to adjust to hair loss.

The impact of my diagnosis has been great on my life and the life of my family members. It's hard having the surgery, chemo, and radiation, and watching your family and friends trying to deal with it. They worry about me constantly and I hate to be a burden, although I know they don't think of me that way. One day you are going along in life and the next you're dealing with a life-threatening disease. You live

with the fear of recurrence. Thank God I continue to be active in my life.
I can't allow this disease to rule my life.

The end of the chemotherapy can also be a difficult time for some women. Did it work? Is all the cancer gone? You no longer have the regular visits to the hospital or treatment center. You may wonder, "Is my body working for me now?" The answer is yes, but it will take time to adjust. You may not feel like yourself again for a few months. You will gradually regain your energy. If you were experiencing depression, this will lift. Your hair will grow back. You will shed the bloating and your complexion will return to normal. If you were experiencing memory loss, this will probably change (for the better!). Food will taste right again. You'll find you now crave foods you could never eat before. You are yourself again, but changed.

Since my treatment ended, I've learned to enjoy myself and to think of
myself. For the first time in my life I'm also spending my money on myself.
Before I thought of my family and spouse first—no more Mrs. Nice Guy.

RADIATION SIDE EFFECTS
Radiation treatments, used as a local treatment after a lumpectomy or mastectomy, are usually given every day for four to six weeks, although this will vary from center to center.

My radiation oncologist recommended that I go back to work immediately
after treatments. My work is very stressful. I said he could go do it, but
I'm taking care of me first.

Daily trips to the hospital or cancer center can be tiring and stressful. Radiation itself will drain the body's energy, leaving you feeling generally weak and tired. The skin around the area receiving radiation may begin to look tanned or sunburned. It may even peel as a result of the burn. It may become very dry or very moist. Your breast may be tender and aching.

You may find that a soft, old, supportive bra, which is not tight, or a loose camisole or T-shirt is most comfortable (not wearing a bra can increase the pain and discomfort). If you did not have a mastectomy, you may notice that your treated breast has changed and become firmer than before. It usually takes about a year after radiation is over for your breast to feel and look normal again. In some cases these changes may last longer and should be checked by you and your doctor. Some women also experience lymphedema as a result of surgery or radiation to the lymph nodes.

It's been five months since I learned I had breast cancer and I am still in radiation therapy. It's taking too long. When it started I felt strong and confident. Now I am depressed and resentful.

HORMONE TREATMENT SIDE EFFECTS

Hormone treatments, like tamoxifen (Nolvadex), are used to treat tumors that are sensitive to hormones. Tamoxifen is given as a pill. Side effects may include weight gain, hot flashes, mood swings, vaginal dryness, changes in your vision, and nausea for the first month. Tamoxifen use has been linked to endometrial cancer and blood clots in rare cases. There is now good evidence from randomized trials that the optimal duration for tamoxifen treatment is five years. You and your doctor should monitor the effects throughout your treatment. You may also want to discuss the newer kinds of hormone treatment drugs, called aromatase inhibitors, that are now being used in the treatment of metastatic breast cancer and, in some instances, early stage breast cancer.

The side effects of tamoxifen are a pain to deal with. However, in the final analysis, they are a small price to pay. I am healthy, disease free, and very much alive.

Things you can learn from a dog:

- Never pass up the opportunity for a joyride.
- Allow the experience of fresh air and wind in your face to be pure ecstasy.
- When the loved ones come home, run to greet them.
- When it's in your best interest, practice obedience.
- Take naps and stretch before rising.
- Romp and play daily.
- Eat with gusto.
- Be loyal.
- Never pretend to be something that you're not.
- If you want what lies buried, dig until you find it.
- When someone is having a bad day, be silent, sit close by, and nuzzle them gently.
- Thrive on attention and let people touch you.
- Avoid biting when a simple growl will do.
- On hot days, drink lots of water and lay under a shady tree.
- When you're happy, dance around and wag your whole body.
- Bond with your pack.
- Delight in the simple joys of a long walk.

—PATTY WOOTEN,

Registered Nurse,

reprinted from *Jest for the Health of It*

Looking after Yourself during Treatment

NUTRITION

When you are going through treatment for breast cancer, maintaining a healthy lifestyle, including diet and exercise, can help you complete the treatment schedule. Good nutrition will help you:

- maintain your strength and minimize tiredness
- rebuild tissue that is damaged by treatment
- fight possible infection

A balanced diet includes choices from each of the food groups: breads and grains, fruits, vegetables, meats and alternatives, and dairy. You may need to eat more high-protein foods to have the energy to meet the demands of treatments.

EMOTIONAL HEALTH

Your treatment period can be lonely and tiring. It is a time when it is more important than ever to be kind to yourself and put your needs first. For some women this isn't always easy. The demands of our personal and work lives are often hard to just put aside for an indefinite period of time. Tell those around you that it is important for you to slow down and rest while you are going through treatment. Learn to ask for help. You may be surprised at how understanding people can be.

"Have I changed? I had such resolutions. And still do, but I have returned to most of my ruts. Yet sometimes, I break out, just for a minute. I do for me, more often, I am more selfish. I enjoy the minutes more. Sometimes."

—BARB SULLIVAN,
My Broken Breast Book

Here are some suggestions for looking after yourself:

- Accept help from "supporters," whomever they may be. Try to pass on work to others who offer to help out.
- Feed your emotional side. This may be through music, books, learning about a new philosophy of life, or whatever gives you

pleasure. Different things work for different people. If you can, don't deny yourself the small things like a warm bath, candles at dinner, or time to be alone or with friends.

- Watch a funny movie or read a funny book. Laughter helps to relax muscles and lift sadness. Learn to play, blow bubbles, laugh, sing, or dance.
- Eat well. Even though you have less of an appetite when you are going through treatment, it is a particularly important time to get the nutrients you need because your body is under added stress. If your appetite is not good, try eating small portions more frequently and eat only when you are feeling well enough to do so. Taking a ten- to fifteen-minute walk before eating helps to increase the appetite.
- Eating well usually requires time for food preparation. If you are the one who usually does the cooking, try to get help from others from time to time. As much as possible, include fruits, vegetables, and grains in what you eat. Try to avoid foods that are hard to digest, such as fried foods, rich sauces or a lot of meat.
- If your mouth is sore from treatment, avoid spicy, salty, and acidic foods, as well as foods that are very hot or cold. Try softer foods such as cooked cereals, yogurt, bananas, applesauce, mashed potatoes, rice, milkshakes, or scrambled eggs. Mouth sores can also be relieved by over-the-counter medications (ask your pharmacist) or by rubbing the contents of a capsule of vitamin E on the sores daily.
- Take time to rest. If you can, give in to a morning or afternoon nap. Go to bed early. Sleep in as much as possible.
- Give yourself permission to listen to your body. It is going through a lot at this time. Listen to what it needs. Go for a walk, drink more water, get a massage, talk to someone who cares about you.
- Some women find keeping a journal to be very therapeutic. Even if you have never done this before, you may find it helpful to write

about what you are going through. It may also help you later to go through your journal to see how you got through such a difficult time.

- If you haven't already done so, consider attending a breast cancer support group meeting. Talking with other women who are going through the same experience can be helpful. Check the Resources section for a group in your area.
- Allow yourself some treats from time to time. You deserve them!
- Deal with your anger constructively. Punch pillows, scream, let your anger out where it isn't going to hurt someone you care about.

When undergoing treatment, some women have found information provided by the Look Good, Feel Better Program to be helpful. See the Resources section at the back of this book for information about how to find the program in your area. Many cancer patients find comfort and spiritual support by focusing attention on the important relationships between themselves and their family, friends, co-workers, church, and community.

"Every moment that I could manage, I was out there marveling over the frothing silk petals of the peonies, the delicately elaborate greenery of the Jacob's Ladder, the graceful swoop and bend of the wild Solomon Seal . . . after a difficult treatment, or a particularly heart-breaking sojourn in the crowded waiting room of sick women, nothing would solace me more than a quick stop at the nursery . . . This year, with spring and regained health, I was doubly and richly rewarded; I'm astonished at how much I tilled and worked and planted, and how much beauty has come rushing back to delight me. I am grateful to the garden."

—MICHELLE LANDSBERG,
The Toronto Star, May 27, 1995

SUMMARY

Your health care team and breast cancer survivors have the experience needed to help you cope with the discomforts of treatment. Family and friends can also be sources of great support, strength, and encouragement. Let them know how you feel, what you need, and when your needs change. No one who cares for you wants to see you suffering. Let others support you.

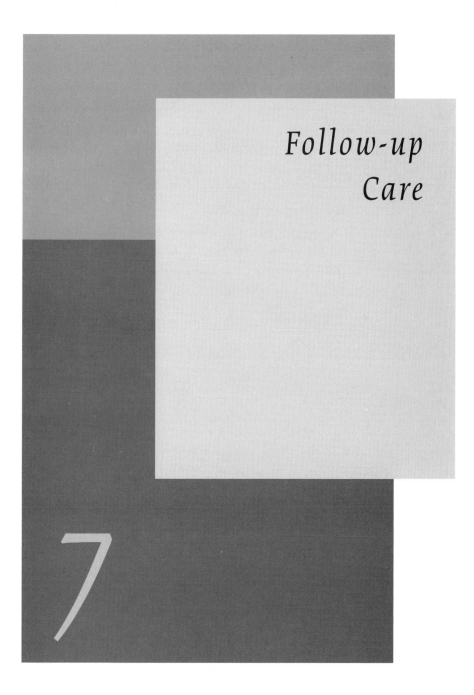

Follow-up Care

7

This chapter is about the emotional and practical realities of getting on with life after your treatments are over. It also provides information about the different kinds of surgery and implants that can be used to reconstruct breast tissue. Not all women choose to have breast reconstruction and many find they are comfortable with one breast or no breast. These choices may be made at any time from the point of diagnosis until years and years after treatment ends.

Sleeping Beauty was awakened by Prince Charming. It took cancer for me to step out of my lethargy. My priorities changed. I realized the urgency and importance of taking my life into my own hands, to live according to my desires, to go and get what I need, and not to accept what I do not want to. Cancer has given me a taste for life—a passionate one.

What to Expect after Your Treatment Ends

Your follow-up care will depend on the type of treatment you have and the region you live in. Usually, after your chemotherapy or radiation is over, or after surgery and recovery, you will see your family doctor, surgeon, and/or oncologist every three to twelve months for the first two years. After two years, you will probably have appointments once every four to twelve months for the following three years. Note that during this period (the first five years after diagnosis) it is necessary to be attended by only one doctor (family physician, surgeon, or oncologist). Choose the one you are most comfortable with. After five years, you should have an annual checkup with your family doctor. Your doctor should ask how you are coping and about any physical changes. He or she will probably order blood tests and a mammogram and do a breast exam. Some doctors will order a chest x-ray. You should also see your family doctor for a regular Pap test and pelvic exam.

If you have not already been shown how to do a skillful breast self-examination (BSE), ask your doctor to show you how or to refer you to someone who can. You may also want to show your doctor how you do a BSE to make sure you are doing it right, especially because of the changes your body has been through. Learn to also examine your scar tissue for any changes.

You should also have a mammogram on an annual basis. If possible, you should have your mammogram done at the same clinic or hospital each time, or ask that your previous mammograms be transferred so they are available for comparison. If you had a breast reconstruction with implants, tell the technologist doing the mammogram. Ask if he or she is experienced doing imaging (x-rays) on implanted breasts.

Some women aren't emotionally prepared for how difficult their annual checkup can be. The uncertainty of knowing whether your cancer has come back can be very distressing. It might be helpful to talk to someone who has already been through this. Bring along someone you trust to these appointments if it will make you feel more comfortable and reassured.

> *Except for the fear of recurrence, especially around mammography time, the quality of my life is the same as it was, maybe even better.*

You may still feel sad after treatment ends. The sadness can be due to a sense of grief or loss, especially if you had a mastectomy. We all grieve in different ways and at our own pace. The sadness, the crying, and the depression will eventually be replaced by a fierce hope and the newfound joy in such simple things as a sunrise or the company of a good friend.

> *Losses were small in terms of transient discomfort and appearance. Many gains were learning to live more fully and openly. I have a better quality*

of life now—no time for pettiness, gossip, complainers. I am content with
what I have and enjoy life to the fullest. I do everything I want to do.

Breast Reconstruction and Prostheses

Today, many women's treatment involves breast-conserving surgery such as a lumpectomy. This means that most of the breast is saved. However, if you had a mastectomy, you may want to consider breast reconstruction.

An estimated two million American women and a half million Canadian women are living with breast cancer. Society is starting to adjust to our one-breasted presence! Still, for other women, replacing their lost breast is worth the discomfort of facing another surgery. Approximately 20 percent of women who have mastectomy surgery will choose to have reconstruction. Some women will have reconstructive surgery at the same time or very soon after a mastectomy. Others will wait for many years before they decide. The choice is up to you.

I was only thirty-five when I lost my breast. After becoming an activist, I
saw my mastectomy scar as a badge of courage—the mark of the Amazon
warrior that I had become. I spent ten years working as an advocate
in Canada and the U.S. in the late 1980s and through the 1990s when
breast cancer wasn't trendy and we had to be brave pioneers. My
daughters were so little when I was diagnosed that they didn't know me
any other way. When they got older, they would ask me to change
where no one could see me at the YMCA pool. As I grew older, I grew
tired of always being a warrior. After the reconstruction, everyone
wanted to know, "How come now and not before?" I couldn't say why,
but the time had come for me to be a plain, old, smart, sexy woman-
warrior—just like everyone else.

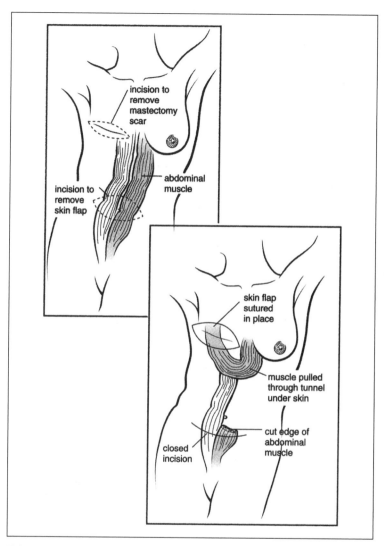

FIGURE 7.1 *Reconstruction using your own tissue involves moving living muscle from the lower abdomen to the area of the mastectomy scar.*

In the past decade, the methods for breast reconstruction have greatly improved. Although a reconstructed breast will never look or feel exactly like your original breast, nor ever be able to make milk or have a nipple that becomes erect, the results can be very good.

There are two types of breast reconstruction. One involves using pieces of the woman's own tissue (sometimes called "flaps") from elsewhere on her body; the other uses implants (Figures 7.1 and 7.2). There are risks associated with each type.

Breast Implants

Breast implants are made of a silicone shell that contains a sterile water-based solution. The implant is placed behind the muscle or breast tissue; therefore it does not make it harder to discover another lump, should the cancer return. You will be able to do breast self-examination and have a mammogram.

The risks of having a surgical implant are the possibility that the scar will become infected or that the implant will fail—that is, it may become hard or the tissue over it may shrink. There has been some controversy in recent years over the long-term safety of silicone breast implants. If you would like to read more about this, see the Resources section on page 142.

> *I do not dwell on the diagnosis. At times there is an overwhelming feeling of "why me?" But having the implants made all the difference to me.*

Breast Reconstruction

If you want breast reconstruction, discuss it with your surgeon and oncologist before your first surgery. It is important to remember that breast reconstruction is major surgery. It is better to have the reconstruction after completing radiation or chemotherapy so it doesn't interfere with your treatment. It may be possible for your surgeon and

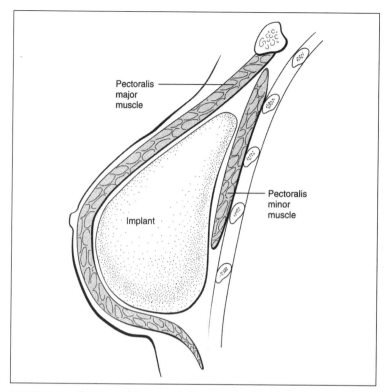

Pectoralis
major
muscle

Pectoralis
minor
muscle

Implant

FIGURE 7.2   *Placement of the internal silicone implant under the chest*

plastic surgeon to do both procedures at the same time, but they are usually done separately. Breast reconstruction is almost always possible after mastectomy. In both the U.S. and Canada, it is fully covered by health insurance plans.

> *Reconstruction has been one of the great joys of my life. I really feel that*
> *my recovery didn't truly begin until I had reconstruction. I marvel at*
> *the "magic of science" and feel blessed to have had access to the best and*
> *most talented specialists in this field. My only regret is that I didn't have*
> *a bilateral!*

How Do I Buy a Prosthesis?

Many women who have had a mastectomy will choose to wear a breast prosthesis (see Figure 7.3). In the early recovery period after your surgery, it is best to wear a lightweight prosthesis to avoid putting any pressure on the scar and surrounding tissue. This is usually made of fabric or foam and covered with a light, stretchy material. Once your healing is further along, you may choose a more permanent breast form. Prostheses are made to be comfortable and look and feel natural. If you can, speak with someone who has already been through this to recommend a good prosthesis fitter in your area. She may also be able to offer you advice on when to buy your prosthesis.

> *I used a prosthesis in my bra for three years but then decided to remake the breast with the use of abdominal muscle. I am happy.*

Usually, your scar is healed enough after a few weeks to wear a prosthesis, which you can buy from a mastectomy boutique or prosthesis fitter. Look in the Resources section on page 142 or under "breast prosthesis" in the telephone directory, or ask the local unit of the American Cancer Society or Canadian Cancer Society. Most fitters require an appointment, which will take about an hour. You might want to ask your husband, partner, or a friend to come with you to the appointment.

> *We have come a long way in twenty-seven years! When I had cancer I had nobody to talk to. I lost both my breasts and my ovaries in one year. My two boys were four and six years old. We had just moved into our house and money was tight. I made my prosthesis from an old bra filled with birdseed and sand. For more than twenty years I have been a volunteer with the Reach for Recovery program and have learned a lot from the couple of hundred women I have seen. All are different.*

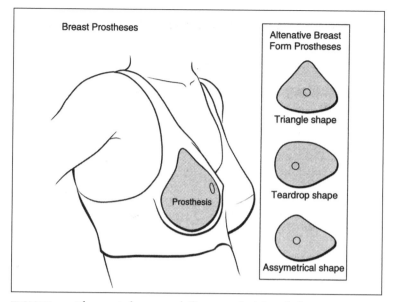

Breast Prostheses

Altenative Breast Form Prostheses

Triangle shape

Teardrop shape

Prosthesis

Assymetrical shape

FIGURE 7.3   *Placement of an external silicone prosthesis into the bra*

Permanent prostheses are more realistic and may be made of polyester, foam rubber, or a soft flesh-like material containing liquid or silicone gel. A prosthesis is designed to weigh the same as normal breast tissue, so when you wear it you won't feel lopsided or have back and shoulder pain. The prosthesis may seem heavy at first and may take some getting used to. It will also warm to your body temperature even though it may feel cold at first.

Mastectomy boutiques also sell bras with a pocket of fabric to hold your prosthesis in place, as well as bathing suits with a bra lining that has a prosthesis pocket. A properly fitted prosthesis should not move around, rub, or irritate your skin. Once in place, you should be able to forget it is there. If you have problems or feel discomfort, go back to your fitter for an adjustment or replacement.

Some government health insurance plans pay for a certain percentage of the prosthesis cost. Group or private insurance plans may cover the rest. Check with your local breast cancer support group, or the government health insurance plan.

Hormone Replacement Therapy and Breast Cancer

If you are experiencing hot flashes and other menopausal symptoms, you should probably not use hormone replacement therapy (HRT). Researchers know that estrogen plays a role in the development of breast cancer. Studies using animals have shown a link between higher levels of estrogen and breast cancer growth. Other studies have shown that women exposed to more estrogen throughout life—for example, women who begin their periods at an early age or enter menopause at a late age—have a higher risk of developing breast cancer. Studies have also shown that women who have never had breast cancer increase their risk of developing the disease if they take HRT for an extended period. The risk of breast cancer increases for each year of use. Furthermore, a woman who has had breast cancer is at risk of having the cancer return or of developing cancer in the opposite breast, and the exposure to estrogen through HRT could trigger the recurrence of breast cancer.

At present, too few studies of HRT use by breast cancer patients have been completed, and the study results available do not indicate that HRT is safe for women who have had breast cancer.

Alternatives to HRT

Several alternative treatments have been studied and found to relieve menopausal symptoms:

- *Hot flashes:* Venlafaxine, a relatively new antidepressant medication marketed as Effexor
- *Vaginal dryness:* K-Y lubricating jelly and Replens, a vaginal moisturizer
- *Sexual and urinary problems:* Estradiol vaginal rings such as Estring, which provide controlled local delivery of very low doses of estrogen (creams are *not* recommended because the estrogen in them passes into the blood, and this can lead to high concentrations of estrogen in the body)

Other alternative treatments have been found to improve bone mass and reduce the risk of osteoporosis:

- exercise, a diet rich in calcium, and appropriate mineral and vitamin supplements
- bone-strengthening drugs called bisphosphonates

One drug used to treat osteoporosis that is *not* recommended for women who have had breast cancer is raloxifene, a selective estrogen receptor modulator. Although it is similar to tamoxifen, a drug commonly used in the treatment of breast cancer, there are no studies supporting raloxifene's use by women with breast cancer.

Other alternative treatments include acupuncture, herbs, and vitamins. Again, there is insufficient evidence to determine effectiveness.

If your menopausal symptoms are particularly troublesome and they are not relieved by any of the alternative approaches listed here, you might still want to discuss HRT with your doctor. You will need to talk about many things, including when you had cancer, what kind of cancer you had, and how your cancer was treated. You will need to weigh your risk of developing a recurrence of breast cancer against your present discomfort. If you decide to use HRT, your doctor will probably suggest a low dosage and short treatment period.

SUMMARY

The physical and emotional stress of treatment is a lot to handle. You'll probably find yourself wondering: "Did it work? Now what?" After treatment ends, your doctor will watch you carefully. You'll be given a follow-up plan for regular visits, blood tests, and mammograms or other imaging tests—depending on your situation. Be sure to report new symptoms or side effects so they can be evaluated and treated.

Intimacy and Relationships

8

When a woman is diagnosed with breast cancer, her husband, lover, or partner can help contribute in many ways to her emotional healing. This chapter is for you and your husband, lover, or partner to read together. It will help you learn how to help each other through this experience.

> *Breast cancer has been a gift. I have learned to say "I." I have learned to say "no." Even though I lost a breast I feel more whole than when I had both breasts.*

Staying Connected

Like other serious illnesses, cancer can bring couples closer, but it can also challenge even the best relationships. Learning how to talk and listen to one another—without being defensive or judgmental—can help your relationship to survive, and even grow, in this difficult time. Whether it is your husband, your lover, or your partner, his or her experience of cancer and yours are not the same. That person is afraid of losing you, afraid that you are suffering. But he or she may also feel pressure to be "strong," to "hold the family together."

> *It is very important to educate the husband that what a woman needs in these times is love. He should meet with the doctor to really know what his wife is going through.*

Both of you may be trying to understand the complex issues of treatment and diagnosis at the same time as you are dealing with your own reactions and emotions. There are ways you can learn to cope with your feelings and still provide emotional and practical help for each other. You can cope by:

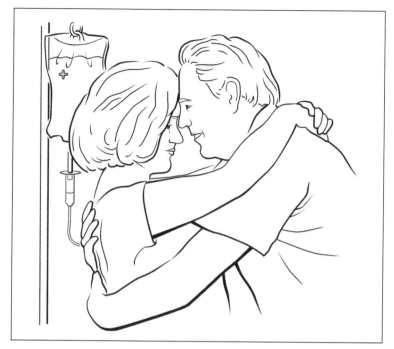

FIGURE 8.1   *Intimacy after breast cancer*

- going together to the doctor's appointments and asking questions;
- keeping a record of questions and the answers;
- keeping a journal of your thoughts and feelings;
- attending a support group for couples or information sessions at your cancer treatment center (call the American Cancer Society or the Canadian Cancer Society for more information);
- talking with other people who have had similar experiences;
- keeping up a program of regular exercise, bodywork, or Tai Chi;
- escaping from the intense pressure of "having cancer" by reading, listening to music, watching movies, enjoying restaurant dinners, or visiting friends;
- making plans for your future;
- trying meditation, prayer, and guided imagery.

I left my spouse because I could not stand his indifference. I felt as though I was living by myself and felt very lonely. He never took care of me. I'm happier now.

FOR HUSBANDS AND PARTNERS

Your wife or partner may be struggling with feelings of fear, anger, depression, and vulnerability, and a sense of being "out of control." Let her know that she can share these feelings with you, that they are not "right" or "wrong," and that you want to know what she is feeling and thinking about. Listen without judging her or trying to provide answers or assurances that "everything is fine." You both know cancer is not "fine"—false assurances don't help. But listening, being support-ive, and helping to understand the disease and its treatments will help her regain confidence in the here and now and maintain hope for your future together.

At first, my husband was great. Now he doesn't even want to talk about it. It's like he's pretending it's not happening!

Many women find they need to talk about breast cancer for a lot longer than their families and friends want to hear about it. And they may fear that they will be abandoned if they are too needy, too demanding of support. One solution is to talk to other women in a support group.

I just got married in April. I have never been married before and have no children. We were hoping there might be a chance we could have at least one. Then I find out I have cancer. It has been a heavy financial burden, and since half of my husband's wages go to child support payments, I need to work. This has added more stress. But I have a very gentle, loving, and understanding husband, who has helped me

through this more than anyone. I feel your partner's attitude toward
you makes a big difference in the healing process. I wouldn't be getting
through this so well without my husband's love and support. He makes
me feel like a whole person.

If I ever wondered what my husband's responses to a medical crisis would
be, I don't have to worry anymore: his support has been outstanding. If a
terrible event can have a positive side, it is this: we are closer than ever.

SEX AFTER BREAST CANCER

For some women, breast cancer will bring no change in their sexual
feelings. Others will find their sexuality enhanced as a result of such a
life-transforming experience. Still others have a temporary lack of sexual desire because of the effects of their treatment or because they do
not feel comfortable with their changed body. And some women may
never have considered sexuality as an important part of their lives and
may consider it even less so after breast cancer.

Stress, worry, anesthesia, pain, radiation and chemotherapy, feeling
ill, and being tired are all powerful depressants, and any depressant is
likely to reduce sexual desire. Generally, if sex was good before, it will
be good again. "Again" frequently comes a few months after the end of
your treatment, about the time that your body stops feeling like someone else's and starts to feel more like home.

My husband and I both had cancer surgery within six months of each
other; he had his penis removed and I lost a breast. What a pair of
"bookends" we made! He died three years ago of a heart attack. Our
sense of humor got us that far.

It is also true that sex has as much to do with the mind as the
body—and everything to do with the heart. At first you may feel shy

or fear rejection; you may want to wear your prosthesis and bra and nightgown and robe to bed. A good, kind, and patient lover loves you, not just one of your breasts. Your lover is waiting for some sort of signal from you that you're ready to make love again. That lovemaking may not set off any fireworks, but then, did you expect it to every time before? Not having a breast, or part of a breast, may mean a few changes in what you're used to doing. But then, you may discover areas of excitement you didn't suspect you had. A good time in bed isn't just for women with two all-natural breasts, or beautiful people, or young people. Good sex is for people who want it enough to make it happen.

How Much Should I Tell My Children or Grandchildren?

Even very young children know when something is wrong. Pretending that everything is normal only increases their fears. It is much kinder to share what you know in a way that they can understand. A very young child can be told that your breast was sick and you had to have an operation, and now you have to take medicine that makes you very tired. This gives the child a chance to help you, for example, by playing quietly while you rest. It also gives the child an opportunity to talk about his or her own fears that you are sick, and that you may go to the hospital. This kind of talking makes it easier for both mother and child to be able to admit to being frightened and uncertain.

Younger children often worry about two things:

- *Who is going to take care of me?* They need to feel safe and protected. They need to know somebody will take care of them.
- *Is mommy going to die?* Be honest with your children and don't make promises that you aren't sure you can keep. Be hopeful and realistic:

"I can't say exactly what will happen to me, but I'm taking medicines that can help me get better. I'm working with the doctors to get better as soon as possible."

Try to maintain some of your normal routine and create the sense of safety and caring that will help them adjust. Tell them honestly about the changes that may happen to your appearance. Encourage them to express their feelings by drawing or singing.

Older children may be angry, or may withdraw. But often, when they know what the problem is and that they are safe, they feel free to talk about their fears. They may also be able to help out around the house, which can help them feel they are contributing to your recovery.

If they don't feel comfortable talking about their fears with you, they can talk to someone else. Cancer is now so common that many children and teens are able to get information and support from friends who have experienced cancer in their own families. Your child's teachers, a school nurse, or cancer center support groups may have information about support services for children. You may find it helpful to talk to your oncologist about your children's reactions to your diagnosis. Often the oncologist can bring a member of your treatment team, such as an experienced nurse or social worker, to talk with your children about cancer.

My children had a lot of trouble coping with me being ill. In hindsight, they probably should have gone to a Kids Can Cope program.

If your children are adults, they may have concerns about their own health. Daughters in particular may be worried about their risk of developing breast cancer. Teenage daughters, for example, may express anger and resentment toward a sick mother. Share this book with them and encourage them to find out more about their own risks. Encourage your adult daughters to do breast self-examinations and, when appropriate, to get routine mammograms. In some cities, breast cancer support groups offer support and information for adult children of people who have had cancer.

Breast Cancer and Pregnancy

If you have been successfully treated for breast cancer, is it okay to get pregnant? Will the treatment harm either you or your baby?

Babies born to women who have had breast cancer are as normal and healthy as those born to women who have never been diagnosed. But receiving treatments (radiation or chemotherapy) while pregnant may cause problems for the baby. Some doctors feel that postponing pregnancy for two years or so after being treated will make it less likely that your cancer will come back. If you are interested in becoming pregnant, it is a good idea to discuss it with your doctor first.

Other Big Cs

Cancer has often been called the "Big C." There are other big Cs.

- *Control* is taking an active part in your care and survival. Control involves sorting out your priorities in life and making choices to give you the greatest possible chance of long-term survival.

- *Compassion* for yourself, first and foremost, is essential. As women, we spend most of our time looking after others. As someone's wife, lover, mother, daughter, sister, neighbor, helper, employer, or employee, we are always serving the needs of others. Now your needs must come first.

I've slowed down and relaxed a lot. I no longer try to perform at the 250 percent rate. One hundred percent is now good enough for me.

Compassion is also for the people who share your life. Although they do not have cancer, they too may be grieving because you have changed. You may not have as much time and energy for them as you did. They may be terrified of having to face a future without you.

- *Communication* may change in your relationships. Cancer places heavy demands on relationships and strains communication. Good relationships may stay good, and even improve. Troubled relationships may get overburdened under the crisis. Cancer doesn't cause divorce. It doesn't cause kids to leave home. But poor communication does cause additional and unnecessary suffering.

When the person who has been the family nurturer suddenly becomes the one most in need of support and care, it is a big change. Roles have shifted. Unwritten rules have changed. And for families unable to talk openly and respectfully, there will be trouble and pain.

You may have to ask for the help you need. You may have to give up some basic household tasks, reduce your work hours (inside or outside your home), and say no to requests for volunteering. You may have to make caring of you your full-time job right now.

I have had a very bad five years. My husband had a bad stroke and I had to look after him. At the same time, I broke my ankle and arm—and found the lump. My main concern was looking after my husband and I worried about what would happen to him if I died. He passed away in May. I'm still going to the clinic that has been so kind to me and I love them all.

SUMMARY

Remember that, like your body, your emotional reaction to treatment will be unique. No one can predict how your cancer will respond to treatment.

Statistics paint an overall picture for everyone diagnosed with the disease. But you may have special strengths—good health, a strong immune system, strong support from family and friends, or a deep spiritual faith—that will help you cope.

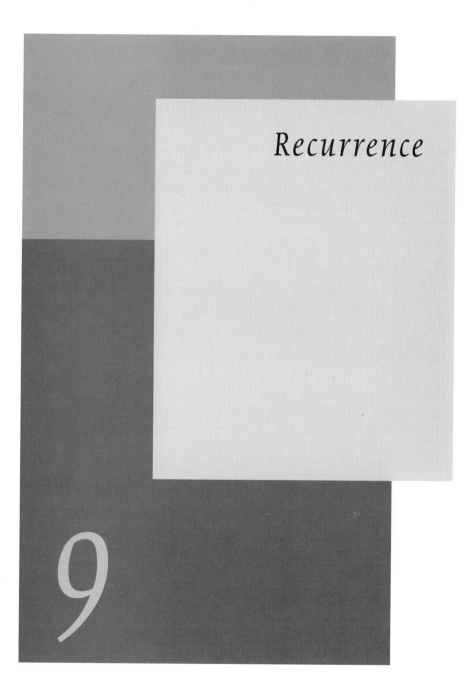

Recurrence

9

This chapter will help you understand your options in the case of recurrence.

> *When I first discovered I had breast cancer my surgeon said I had a 75 percent chance of recovery. When the cancer recurred, I knew I would make it again. I was put on tamoxifen and then megace. I am now having chemotherapy and I know it is helping me. My outlook is very positive.*

What if the Cancer Comes Back?

It is a terrible shock to learn that the cancer is back. It brings the same fear, anger, and pain as it did before. It also brings a feeling that somehow you have failed. Did you not fight the cancer hard enough? Or not have treatment for long enough? Or choose the wrong treatment, the wrong caregivers?

The difference this time is that you have taken this trip before. You've traveled through cancer territory and faced its difficulties and challenges. You can do it again.

> *I was devastated and traumatized by the original misdiagnosis. Chemotherapy was truly dreadful, and I suffered with it for a full two years. Ten years later chemotherapy was much better due to effective antinauseants. I was thrilled to have the opportunity to have a bone marrow transplant, and the stress was worth it. My cancer has recurred once again and, except for being concerned about my children, who are suffering, I am living with it quite well.*

This recurrence may be a new cancer, but more likely it is a few cells that have broken away from your breast and traveled through your lymph system or bloodstream to a new site in your body. This cancer is called "metastatic disease," or you may hear people say your cancer has "metastasized." This would be the same type of cancer as the original. If, for example, it is in your liver, it is not liver cancer; it is breast cancer that has spread to your liver. Recurrence can also be local, in or around the mastectomy scar or in the breast that had the lumpectomy, or regional, in the lymph nodes under the arm or in the shoulder near the breast that had cancer.

> *My first experience with cancer was twenty-seven years ago at age thirty-one. Emotionally, I went from one extreme to the other. The first time, nothing was going to get in my way. My second experience—a mastectomy—was very sobering and brought me to a new level of maturity and a new way of seeing myself in relation to the world around me. The third or fourth time around I went into a year of depression and anxiety, which produced my greatest learning experience: to face reality and take care of myself emotionally and physically. I made more positive changes in my relationships and lifestyle when I emerged from this period. I kept a diary of my feelings, which taught me a lot about myself when I was finally able to read it. I always thought it could be helpful to share it with someone going through the same thing. In some ways, this period of self-examination was worse than cancer.*

Treatments for cancer recurrence are the same as the first occurrence: surgery, radiation, chemotherapy, and hormone therapy. Researchers are currently studying new forms of chemotherapy and biological therapies. Your choice of treatment depends on what kind of treatments you had before, how much your cancer responds to hormones (its hormone receptor levels), how long has passed between your first treatments and the recurrence, the site of recurrence, and whether or not you have gone through menopause. As always, the aim of the treatment will be to control the cancer while simultaneously maximizing the quality of life.

> *The quality of life is still good. I'm a better person, more sensitive to others, more understanding, kinder, and more loving. My spiritual life is stronger and I have no fear of death, but I do want my suffering eased as much as possible.*

There are a number of drugs available to treat breast cancer recurrence. Hormone drugs include tamoxifen, megace, and aromatese inhibitors such as anastrozole (Arimidex), letrozole (Femora), and exemestane (Aromasin). There are many chemotherapy drugs. Some have been around longer than others and more is known about them. One commonly used drug in the United States and Canada is doxorubicin (Adriamycin). Other drugs that are now available include paclitaxel (Taxol), docetaxel (Taxotere), vinorelbine (Navelbine), epirubicin (Ellence) and capecitabine (Xeloda). These drugs have been approved for treating metastatic disease that doesn't respond to standard chemotherapy. However, they are not a cure for breast cancer. Some women cannot tolerate these drugs at all, but for others they have improved their lives. Other drugs currently being researched are also showing some promise for women with metastatic breast cancer. Ask your oncologist what he or she knows about these drugs and whether they might be appropriate for you. There are also many trials for women with recurrence. This is something you should discuss with your doctor.

> "What is there possibly left for us to be afraid of, after we have dealt face to face with death and not embraced it? Once I accept the existence of dying, as a life process, who can ever have power over me again?"
>
> —AUDRE LORDE

When women face a poor prognosis, many get very angry. The anger is often over caregivers (doctors, nurses, or family members) ignoring the need for emotional support. Your relationship with your caregivers will depend very much on how comfortable you are talking about your fears, concerns, needs, and hopes. Be specific about what you expect from them. Let them know when you are in pain. Tell them you want to know about *all* the treatment options, and ask about clinical trials that may be underway at other treatment centers. You can also get information from the American Cancer Society in the U.S., or the Cancer Information Service in Canada.

Good listening skills and respect for what you and your family are experiencing can provide comfort and allow you to move through the stages of grief and anger that accompany a life-threatening prognosis. But many caregivers and family members are unable to provide the support needed. If so, the support can often be found in others within the family circle, friends, caregivers, and the community. The palliative care team, hospice program, or bereavement groups in your community can help you and those who care about you through this difficult time. They can help at any time during the progress of the disease, not just at the very end of life. Ask for help when you or someone you care about is suffering. No one needs to suffer alone or without good pain management.

SUMMARY

Remember that there are ways to help you cope with your fears and anxiety in the event of cancer recurrence. A number of treatments—including radiation, hormones, and chemotherapy—are available. The type of treatment chosen will depend on many factors. The goal is to control the cancer while at the same time maximizing quality of life. You can gather information from your caregivers and from the sources listed in the Resources section on page 142. You can contribute to your own care by using the healing techniques that might have helped you in the past. You can call upon those counselors, friends, and family members who helped you in the past, to help renew your strength and spirit again.

Conclusion

Advocates and Activists

This chapter discusses how and why some women choose to be involved in breast cancer advocacy.

This Isn't Fair!

You're right. It shouldn't have happened to you, or any of us, but it has. Maybe you've thought about giving up, about not fighting back. Most of us do at some point. But after the devastation and loneliness pass, when you're not so tired and miserable and sad, you will begin to think of life again. With time you will rediscover the opportunities that life can offer. You will make plans again.

> "Anniversary. A year. I have lived every minute of the day one year ago. I feel again the absolute devastation. Desolation. I want to find a quiet place and cry. But today's life intrudes and I don't have time. This is good. Remember but don't dwell. Life goes on."
>
> —BARB SULLIVAN,
> *My Broken Breast Book*

For some women, recovery from breast cancer involves becoming an advocate. American and Canadian women know that public pressure can influence government commitments to critical health issues. Breast cancer activists are now demanding increased research funding, improved early detection methods, real prevention, and the involvement and influence of survivors in setting the research agenda and influencing all aspects of public policy in breast cancer.

Some women choose to become activists after diagnosis and treatment, or after participating in a support group. For some women, an advocacy group is support—another way of making sense of the experience of surviving breast cancer. A diagnosis of breast cancer profoundly influences a woman's concerns about her future, and that of her daughters and other women she cares about. Activism can provide opportunities for women to make a difference. For women who were activists in the feminist movement or the environmental or consumer movements before their diagnosis, the progression to breast cancer activism may be natural and obvious. You can find contacts for advocacy groups in the U.S. and Canada in the Resources section on page 142.

It is essential to recognize, however, that not all of us will choose to be activists. Some women will avoid it because it involves identifying with cancer. Most women try to forget about cancer as much as possible because they need to feel and be perceived as normal after a cancer diagnosis. Each of us must discover for ourselves what work and which relationships will make our lives meaningful. We must respect the choices each woman makes based on her life experiences, abilities, beliefs, and commitments. The most valued possession each of us has is time. How we choose to spend our time is up to each of us to determine.

Glossary

ANESTHESIA: A drug or gas that is used to remove the feeling of pain. Local anesthesia involves the injection of a drug into a small area before a painful procedure, such as surgery. General anesthesia causes loss of consciousness.

AXILLARY DISSECTION: Axilla is a term used for the armpit. An axillary dissection is surgery that removes some of the lymph nodes in the armpit.

BIOPSY: Removing tissue from some part of the body to study it more closely under a microscope for diagnosis.

BONE MARROW: The soft tissue that is found inside the bones. Red and white blood cells and platelets are produced in the bone marrow.

CARCINOGEN: Any substance that can cause cancer.

CAT SCAN: CAT stands for computerized axial tomography. This is a method of diagnosis that uses computers as well as x-rays. It can study tumors more closely than conventional x-rays.

CHEMOTHERAPY (CHEMO): Treatment that uses drugs to kill cancer cells. The drugs can be in the form of pills or injections.

DNA: Material present in living organisms that carries genetic information.

DUCT: A tube in the body that carries body fluids. In the breast, milk ducts carry milk from the lobule to the nipple. Sometimes cancer can develop in the milk ducts.

DYSPLASIA: Abnormality in development. In disease, any change in the size, shape, and organization of adult cells.

ESTROGEN RECEPTORS: Protein in cancer cells that binds to the female hormone estrogen.

GENES: Genes exist within cells in the body. They are the blueprint of the characteristics we inherit from our parents.

GRADE: A measure of how aggressive cancer cells look under a microscope. The more aggressive the cancer cells look, the more likely they are to spread to other parts of the body.

HORMONES: Chemicals within the body that control growth, reproduction, sexual characteristics, and metabolism. Hormones are secreted into the blood and transported to specific organs (such as the breast).

HYPERPLASIA: The abnormal increase in the number of normal cells in normal arrangement in a tissue.

IN SITU: In the natural or normal place. A tumor that is confined to the site of origin and not invading neighboring tissue. It is not yet a cancer.

INVASIVE: A characteristic of malignant tumors, which invade and actively destroy surrounding tissue. Invasion is what defines a cancer.

LOBULE: Lobes in the breast are divided into smaller structures called lobules. Milk is made in this part of the breast.

LUMPECTOMY: Surgery that removes the cancerous lump or tumor and a small amount of the normal breast tissue around it.

LYMPH: A body fluid that is similar to blood but does not have red blood cells. It transports white blood cells called lymphocytes. The function of the lymph system is to provide fluid to body tissues and to carry waste away from the cells. Lymph flows through the body in the lymph vessels.

LYMPHEDEMA: A swelling of one of the limbs (arm, leg) as a result of the removal or radiation of the lymph nodes and lymph vessels in that limb. In women with breast cancer, this can occur in the arm or hand on the side that the surgery was done. It can occur any time after surgery.

LYMPH NODES: Small lima-bean-shaped structures of the lymph system that act as filters.

MASTECTOMY: Surgery that removes the entire breast that is affected by cancer.

METASTASIS: The spread of cancer to another part of the body. The cancer cells are usually carried by the bloodstream or the lymphatic system.

MRI SCAN: MRI stands for magnetic resonance imaging. It is a technique that transmits radio waves through the body using a magnet and electric coil. A picture is then reconstructed using a computer. MRI scans can provide more detailed information about tumors.

ONCOGENES: Genes that are capable of changing normal cells to cancer cells.

ONCOLOGIST: Oncology is the study of cancer, and an oncologist is a doctor who specializes in treating cancer patients.

PATHOLOGIST: A doctor who specializes in examining body tissues. He or she determines if a disease is present.

PROGNOSIS: An estimate of whether a disease (such as cancer) will stay the same or get worse in the future.

PROSTHESIS: An artificial substitute for a missing part of the body, such as a breast. For breast cancer patients, a breast form made of fabric or silicone that fits into the bra. A prosthesis can be used for both cosmetic or functional reasons (e.g., to ensure normal weight and balance to prevent sore shoulders or back problems).

RADIATION THERAPY: High-energy radiation can be used to treat cancer by damaging and killing cancer cells. It is usually used after surgery if there is a risk that some cancer cells may have been left behind.

RADIOISOTOPES: Radioactive materials given to patients to make the organ that picks it up scannable.

SILICONE: A durable, synthetic substance that is used in some breast implants.

SYSTEMIC THERAPIES: Drug therapies that work throughout your blood system. They may be recommended after your surgery or, in some cases, before. Also referred to as adjuvant systemic therapies, most involve anticancer medication (chemotherapy or hormone therapy) given after surgery to a woman who seems to be at high risk for a recurrence of her cancer. These therapies are also used if cancer recurs.

Breast Cancer Resources

American Cancer Society
Toll-free: 1-800-ACS-2345
Web site: www.cancer.org

American Institute for Cancer Research
1759 R Street N.W.
Washington, DC 20009
Toll-free: 1-800-843-8114
Tel: (202) 328-7744
Fax: (202) 328-7226
E-mail: aicrweb@aicr.org
Web site: www.aicr.org

Look Good . . . Feel Better
Toll-free: 1-800-395-LOOK
Web site:
   www.lookgoodfeelbetter.org

National Alliance of Breast Cancer Organizations (NABCO)
9 East 37th Street, 10th Floor
New York, NY 10016
Toll-free: 1-888-80-NABCO
Web site: www.nabco.org

National Breast Cancer Coalition (NBCC)
1707 L Street, NW, Suite 1060
Washington, D.C. 20036
Toll-free: 1-800-622-2838
Tel: (202) 296-7477
Fax: (202) 265-6854
Web site: www.natlbcc.org

National Cancer Institute
Public Inquiries Office
6116 Executive Boulevard, MSC8322
Suite 3036A
Bethesda, MD 20892-8322
Toll-free: 1-800-4-CANCER
TTY: 1-800-332-8615
Web site: www.nci.nih.gov

National Coalition for Cancer Survivorship (NCCS)
1010 Wayne Avenue, Suite 770
Silver Spring, MD 20910
Toll-free: 1-877-NCCS-YES
Tel: (301) 650-9127
Fax: (301) 565-9670
E-mail: info@canceradvocacy.org
Web site:
   www.canceradvocacy.org

National Lymphedema Network

Latham Square
1611 Telegraph Avenue, Suite 1111
Oakland, CA 94612-2138
Toll-free: 1-800-541-3259
Tel: (510) 208-3200
Fax: (510) 208-3110
E-mail: nln@lymphnet.org
Web site: www.lymphnet.org

National Women's Health Information Center

8550 Arlington Boulevard, Suite 300
Fairfax, VA 22031
Toll-free: 1-800-994-9662
TTY: 1-888-220-5446
Web site: www.4woman.gov

Reach to Recovery

For general inquiries or to receive contact information for your local chapter, call the American Cancer Society
Toll-free: 1-800-ACS-2345

Susan G. Komen Breast Cancer Foundation

5005 LBJ Freeway, Suite 250
Dallas, TX 75244
Toll-free: 1-800-IM-AWARE
Tel: (972) 855-1600
Web site: www.komen.org

U.S. Food and Drug Administration (FDA)

Breast Implant Information Line
Toll-free: 1-800-532-4440

Y-ME National Breast Cancer Association

212 W. Van Buren, Suite 500
Chicago, IL 60607
Toll-free: 1-800-221-2141
Tel: (312) 986-8338
Fax: (312) 294-8597
E-mail: help@y-me.org
Web site: www.y-me.org

CANADA

**Breast Cancer Advocacy
    Canada**
c/o PISCES (Partnering in Self-
    Help Community Education
    & Support)
2046 Grovetree Lane
Burlington, ON L7R 4V4
Tel: (905) 637-2840
Fax: (905) 637-8536
E-mail: pisces1@on.aibn.com
Web site: www.piscesonline.ca

**Breast Cancer Society
    of Canada**
401 St. Clair Street
Point Edward, ON N7V 1P2
Toll-free: 1-800-567-8767
Tel: (519) 336-3710
Fax: (519) 336-6846
E-mail: bcsc@bcsc.ca
Web site: www.bcsc.ca

Breast Implant Line of Canada
56 Touraine Avenue
North York, ON M3H 1R2
Tel: (416) 636-6618
Fax: (416) 636-3570
Web site: www.info-implants.
    com/Ontario/Attis/01.html

**Canadian Breast Cancer
    Foundation**
National Office
790 Bay Street, Suite 1000
Toronto, ON M5G 1N8
Toll-free: 1-800-387-9816
Tel: (416) 596-6773
Fax: (416) 596-7857
Web site: www.cbcf.org

**Canadian Breast Cancer
    Network**
331 Cooper Street, Suite 602
Ottawa, ON K2P 0G5
Toll-free: 1-800-685-8820
Tel: (613) 230-3044
Fax: (613) 230-4424
E-mail: cbcn@cbcn.ca
Web site: www.cbcn.ca

**Canadian Breast Cancer
    Research Initiative**
10 Alcorn Avenue, Suite 200
Toronto, ON M4V 3B1
Tel: (416) 961-9406
Fax: (416) 961-4189
E-mail: cbcri@cancer.ca
Web site: www.breast.cancer.ca

Canadian Cancer Society
National Office
10 Alcorn Avenue, Suite 200
Toronto, ON M4V 3B1
Toll-free: 1-888-939-3333
Tel: (416) 961-7223
Fax: (416) 961-4189
E-mail: info@cis.cancer.ca
Web site: www.cancer.ca

**Cancer Advocacy Coalition
   of Canada**
180 Bloor Street West, Suite 904
Toronto, ON M5S 2V6
Toll-free: 1-877-472-3436
Web site: www.canceradvocacy
   coalition.com

Health Canada
Ottawa, ON K1A 0K9
Tel: (613) 957-2991
Fax: (613) 941-5366
E-mail: info@hc-sc.gc.ca
Web site: www.hc-sc.gc.ca

Hope Air
(formerly Mission Air
   Transportation Network)
Procter & Gamble Building
4711 Yonge Street
Toronto, ON M2N 6K8

Tel: (416) 222-6335
Fax: (416) 222-6930
E-mail: mail@hopeair.org
Web site: www.hopeair.org

Look Good Feel Better (LGFB)
420 Britannia Road East, Suite 102
Mississauga, ON L4Z 3L5
Toll-free: 1-800-914-5665
E-mail: lgfb@lgfb.ca
Web site:
   www.lookgoodfeelbetter.ca

Reach to Recovery
For general inquiries or to
receive contact information for
your local chapter, call the
Canadian Cancer Society's
Cancer Information Service
Toll-free: 1-888-939-3333

**Willow Breast Cancer Support
   and Resource Services**
785 Queen Street East
Toronto, ON M4M 1H5
Toll-free: 1-800-778-3100
Tel: (416) 778-5000
Fax: (416) 778-8070
Web site: www.willow.org

Index